GUTSY

GUTSY

living my best life
with Crohn's disease
& ulcerative colitis

HEATHER
FEGAN

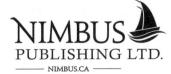

NIMBUS
PUBLISHING LTD.
— NIMBUS.CA —

Nimbus Publishing Limited
3660 Strawberry Hill Street, Halifax, NS, B3K 5A9
(902) 455-4286 nimbus.ca

Printed and bound in Canada
NB1624

"Gutsy" is a trademark of Crohn's and Colitis Canada

Author's disclaimer: While I'm an expert on being a person with Crohn's disease, I am not a healthcare professional. If you have a health concern, please seek professional medical advice.

Editor: Angela Mombourquette

Nimbus Publishing is based in Kjipuktuk, Mi'kma'ki, the traditional territory of the Mi'kmaq People.

Library and Archives Canada Cataloguing in Publication

Title: Gutsy : living my best life with Crohn's disease & ulcerative colitis / Heather Fegan.
Names: Fegan, Heather, author.
Identifiers: Canadiana (print) 2023022217X | Canadiana (ebook) 20230222196 | ISBN 9781774711620 (softcover) ISBN 9781774711637 (EPUB)
Subjects: LCSH: Fegan, Heather—Health. | LCSH: Crohn's disease—Patients—Canada—Biography. | LCSH: Ulcerative colitis—Patients—Canada—Biography. | LCGFT: Autobiographies.
Classification: LCC RC862.E52 F44 2023 | DDC 362.196/3440092—dc23

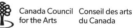

Canada Council   Conseil des arts
for the Arts   du Canada

Nimbus Publishing acknowledges the financial support for its publishing activities from the Government of Canada, the Canada Council for the Arts, and from the Province of Nova Scotia. We are pleased to work in partnership with the Province of Nova Scotia to develop and promote our creative industries for the benefit of all Nova Scotians.

For Matt, Anna, and Rosie, for helping me live my best life.
And to all the fellow IBD patients out there—you are not alone.

CONTENTS

INTRODUCTION

I wrote this book because I wanted to create a gutsy and friendly guide to Crohn's disease and ulcerative colitis that Canadians can relate to—a guide that the hundreds of thousands of people who have been diagnosed with Inflammatory Bowel Disease (IBD) can pick up and learn something from—or just feel inspired. I hope it can also be a resource for those who know and care for people with IBD.

This guide is a memoir of my twenty-five years of living with the disease, anchored with expert interviews, punctuated with facts and statistics, and supported with anecdotal evidence from fellow Crohnies.

Several chapters here explore my personal journey with Crohn's; others include conversations with doctors, nurse practitioners, dietitians, psychologists, and researchers as we explore causes, incidence rates, risk factors, navigating drug coverage, research in IBD, self-advocacy, psychology, and nutrition.

Nova Scotia has the highest prevalence rate per one hundred thousand people of IBD in the country and, given that Canada has one of the highest reported rates of IBD in the world, this means Nova Scotia, where I'm from, has among the highest prevalence of Crohn's and colitis anywhere.

In 2023, approximately 322,600 Canadians—an estimated 1 in 121—are living with IBD. That estimate includes nearly 12,000 people in Nova Scotia. It is more than twice as common as multiple sclerosis or HIV and as prevalent as epilepsy and Type 1 diabetes.

There is no cure and little public understanding of the pain, chronic suffering, and isolation IBD patients courageously cope with every day of their lives. In 2023, IBD is estimated to cost $5.38 billion in combined direct, indirect, and out-of-pocket expenses—an average of $16,676 per patient—and this may be an underestimate of the true financial burden.

People living with IBD face many challenges, including social stigma, anxiety and depression, lack of awareness of IBD as a chronic disease, lack of equity in access to care, and lack of access to expensive IBD medications.

I've had Crohn's for over half my life, have had multiple surgeries, and have been on most of the available treatments for the disease. I have decades of experience with IBD. But while I'm an experienced patient, please keep in mind that I'm not a healthcare professional.

I don't intend to make light of a serious—at times debilitating—condition that affects many Canadians. I do intend to approach these topics in an honest and optimistic, hopeful, and positive manner to prove to people of all ages that they can still live life to the fullest despite their disease.

I'll tell you now that by the time you reach the end of this book you'll see that this story has not ended. My unknowable journey continues, but one thing I can promise is that, true to this book's subtitle, I am genuinely living my best life with Crohn's disease.

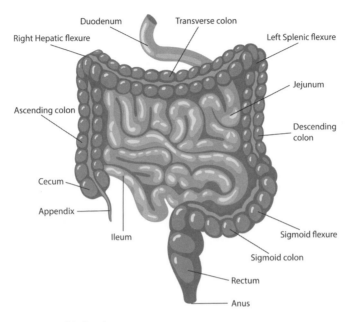

The anatomy of the intestine.

IBD CHEAT SHEET

Inflammatory bowel disease (IBD) describes a group of conditions, the two main forms of which are Crohn's disease and ulcerative colitis. IBD also includes indeterminate colitis (also known as Crohn's colitis).

In a nutshell, IBD causes sections of the gastrointestinal tract to become inflamed and ulcerated. Inflammation in our bodies can be a good thing, it happens when your immune system is fighting a possible threat. But an overactive immune system may attack healthy parts of the body, causing damage to healthy tissue.

CROHN'S DISEASE
PATCHY INFLAMMATION THROUGHOUT
SMALL AND LARGE BOWEL

ULCERATIVE COLITIS
CONTINUOUS AND UNIFORM
INFLAMMATION IN THE LARGE BOWEL

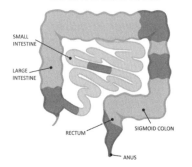
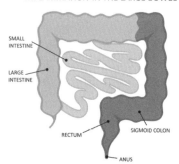

A comparison of Crohn's disease and colitis.

- Inflammation from Crohn's can strike anywhere in the gastrointestinal (GI) tract from mouth to anus but is usually located in the lower part of the small intestine and the upper colon. Patches of inflammation are spread out between healthy portions of the gut and can penetrate the intestinal layers from inner to outer lining.

- Ulcerative colitis is more localized in nature than Crohn's disease. Typically, the disease affects the colon (large intestine) including the rectum and anus, and only invades (inflames) the inner lining of bowel tissue. It almost always starts at the rectum, extending upward in a continuous manner through the colon. Colitis can be controlled with medication and in severe cases can even be treated through the surgical removal of the entire large intestine.

- Indeterminate colitis is a term used when it is unclear if the inflammation is due to Crohn's disease or ulcerative colitis.

Source: crohnsandcolitis.ca/About-Crohn-s-Colitis/
What-are-Crohns-and-Colitis

MY STORY:
FROM DIAGNOSIS
TO COLECTOMY
(1997–2002)

I was fifteen years old when I was diagnosed with ulcerative colitis. It all started with a pain in my side that the doctors thought was appendicitis. The dull ache turned into sharp, stabbing pains across my belly triggered by abdominal contractions that came in waves—wrenching cramps that clenched and tightened every time I ate anything, making me double over in pain. My family doctor referred me to a specialist—Dr. Micheline Ste-Marie, a gastroenterologist—and I had appointments and procedures one after the other, all in an attempt to determine what was causing the pain, the fatigue, the nausea, the vomiting, and the diarrhea. I swallowed barium, a chalky liquid that would show my gastrointestinal tract on an X-ray. I had indium, a radioactive material used in tiny amounts, injected into my body to measure the degree of inflammation in my belly. I had ultrasounds and blood tests, and I was poked and prodded like some sort of specimen in a lab.

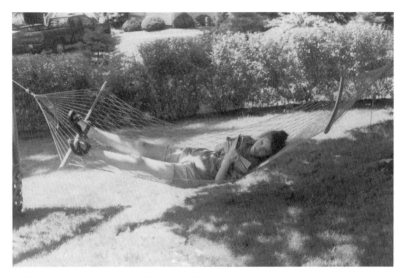

Heather as a teenager before she was diagnosed with inflammatory bowel disease.

January 24, 1998

Dear Diary,

On Wednesday I had to drink 300 ml of this really gross stuff, and again on Thursday where I went to the hospital for a test. They put me to sleep using laughing gas; it was so weird. I was so confused when I woke up! I had to get an IV and now I have a huge bruise on my hand. The doctors don't know what's wrong with me but they found some inflammation in my stomach and are doing more tests. I'm kind of worried about what it is, but probably nothing major…

I remember sitting with my mom in Dr. Ste-Marie's very small rectangular office at the IWK Health Centre (the children's hospital for Atlantic Canada) on Friday, February 6,

1998. All the testing, procedures, and examinations were complete. The office door had opened and Dr. Ste-Marie, a petite older woman with a strong French accent, came in and placed my thick file on her desk.

"Heather," she asked straight away, "have you heard of a disease called ulcerative colitis?" I hadn't, but this was what she had determined I had. It is an illness with no known cause—perhaps a defective gene or an autoimmune disorder—and no known cure. It's a type of chronic inflammatory bowel disease that attacks the digestive system, causing the intestines to become inflamed, form sores, bleed easily, scar, and lose the natural smoothness of their inner lining.

Unlike Crohn's disease, a similar yet distinct condition that can affect any part of the gastrointestinal tract, the symptoms were affecting only my large intestine. Ulcerative colitis affects only the colon, leading Dr. Ste-Marie to the diagnosis.

She explained that some people have their colon removed to eliminate the disease, but she was confident my symptoms could be brought under control with anti-inflammatory drugs.

"If you ever need surgery, your body will let you know when it's time," she said—a valuable piece of advice that has stuck with me since that day. She also warned about the unpredictability of the disease. It could flare up and attack at any moment without warning. It could also seemingly disappear and send a patient into a blissful remission lasting days, weeks, or even years. Dr. Ste-Marie also admitted she wasn't 100 percent certain this was what was wrong with me. "If the disease persists or goes into remission and comes back again, then we will all know for sure."

I listened to everything she said, took it all in, and thought that I understood. She wrote me a prescription for an anti-inflammatory medication, and I didn't think much of it, apart from the fact I was pleased to be receiving something that would finally make me feel better. I was eager to get back to school. My friends and I had important things to discuss during our grade 9 science class—like what to wear to the next school dance.

As sick as I had been feeling, I had made a conscious effort not to let it affect my life. I refused to miss out on anything and continued to go to school, take dance lessons, and hang out with my friends on the weekend. Where my energy came from, I wasn't sure, because I had a total loss of appetite. When I didn't eat, I had no abdominal contractions, no sharp, wrenching cramps. When I didn't eat, I didn't feel any pain.

But by the following Monday, I was so ill I couldn't get out of bed.

"You have to eat something," my mom pleaded for what felt like the hundredth time. My health had rapidly declined over the weekend, plummeting to the lowest point yet. I felt really sick; I was weak and exhausted, the horrible pains now constant. On Tuesday I was still in bed in a dazed sort of trance. My mom and my older sister were hovering over me. They had resorted to temptation now, my sister with a milkshake from the Chickenburger, a local diner, in one hand and a McDonald's Happy Meal in the other. But I couldn't. I knew the food moving through my body would just be too painful. I was running a fever now, so Mom had decided to call the clinic at the IWK.

My dad pushed the wheelchair off the elevator on the seventh floor. I clutched the gym bag resting on my lap even tighter. "Murphy's law," Mom had told me earlier that afternoon. "If we pack a bag and bring it—be prepared—then you won't have to stay." Yeah, right. She probably just didn't want me to panic when she got off the phone with the nurse, who suggested I be brought into the emergency room and to bring a bag, just in case.

The doctors in the emergency room took one look at me and knew I had to be admitted. I'd lost twenty pounds in two weeks; my face, drained of colour, was sunken like a skeleton. I could barely sit up on my own. There was no option other than a hospital admission. At the very least I needed an IV to pump fluids into my body to stop the dehydration.

Now, as I was being wheeled down the hall, the distinct, sterile smell of hospital air nearly suffocating me, I was glad to have that bag with some home comforts inside—my slippers, my own pyjamas, a familiar blanket.

My mom led the way as we followed the signs for Seven East and pushed through two very large swinging doors, entering the general medicine ward. Room nine was on the left, and I double-checked the flimsy green plastic bracelet on my wrist to make sure that was where I was being sent.

We entered the small room to find one of the three beds already occupied. I took one look at the girl sitting on the first bed and my heart started beating faster. She was hooked up to a major contraption. Two IV lines escaped the sleeve of her shirt; another protruded from the back of her hand. The wires twisted and tangled their way to the shiny silver IV pole standing beside her bed. Bags of liquid hung from the top of the pole—big, fat bags with yellow juice, a pouch with clear fluid, and another with what looked like milk. Beneath these, fastened to the pole, was a blue box that beeped and flashed, numbers ticking up and down. Beneath that still, a grey pump, whirring and clicking away. My heart pounded just looking at this machine. I couldn't imagine how the girl felt. Something must be seriously wrong with her.

I forced a timid hello with a polite smile and the girl returned my greeting. My dad brought the wheelchair to a stop in front of the second bed. My name, written on a piece of tape, was stuck to the foot.

I tried to settle into the uncomfortable surroundings of the hospital room with my parents' help. Spread out, my colourful quilt from home helped to brighten the room and counteract all its neutral colours just a little. Drawing the curtains around my bed, I changed out of the stiff, scratchy hospital gown I had put on in the emergency room and into my own cozy pyjamas. A nurse came in and started an IV in the back of my hand; at this point my IV pole held only one bag of clear fluid. She explained a doctor would be in to see me in the morning and suggested I "relax" and get some sleep in the meantime.

My parents had to leave, but before they went, I asked them to open the curtains around my bed. It was claustrophobic, being enclosed in such a tiny space. The other girl also had her curtains drawn back and was tucked into bed, just like me. She looked about my age, and her shoulder-length brown hair looked just like mine. The woman sitting with her introduced herself to my parents. Her name was Victoria, and she was Jamie-Lee's mother. The stand beside Jamie-Lee's bed held a stereo, a picture frame, a box of tissues, and books. It looked like Jamie-Lee had been there for a while, and I felt bad.

"We'll be back first thing in the morning," my mom promised. Victoria left with my parents, and Jamie-Lee and I were left alone. We still hadn't said more than hello to one another. Seconds after they left the room, a nurse poked her head in the door. "Lights out girls; get some rest."

I tugged on the chain hanging beside my bed at the same time Jamie-Lee pulled on hers and the lights went out. After a few moments of silence, her voice came out of the darkness. "Heather, what are you here for?"

"I have something called ulcerative colitis," I responded.

Her reply came instantly: "Oh, that's what I have." My stomach churned. I froze, motionless, as her words echoed in my head. This girl I felt bad for, the one hooked up to the frightening machine who looks like she's lived in this hospital for a while—she has what I have? I couldn't speak another word. Now I was really scared.

March 13, 1998

Dear Diary,

Wow! I haven't written in two months and boy do I have a lot to write about…. It's weird; I always wanted something about me to be different. I wanted there to be something unique about me. Now I have a disease that doesn't have a cure that I'll have forever! I feel better, 100% better. I never realized how sick I was, but it must've been pretty bad, compared to how much better I feel now, and I still don't have all my energy back. People keep asking if I'm better and I just say, yeah, I feel better but I guess they don't know I have and am gonna have colitis forever. And I always assume that they know what it is. I keep forgetting that up until I was diagnosed a month ago, I'd never heard the word in my life before.

I survived that first hospital stay. Like Jamie-Lee, I was hooked up to a contraption of wires and machines that whirred and beeped. Bags of liquid nutrition hung high on my IV pole—total parenteral nutrition (TPN) it was called. The liquid was delivered through a major vein in my chest, bypassing my intestines altogether, allowing my stomach to rest and the inflammation to heal. For three weeks I ate nothing by mouth, and yet was never struck by hunger. The hospital had a classroom, and each morning for an hour and a half volunteer tutors helped me with the work my schoolteachers had faxed over. In the afternoons, I was unhooked from all the tubes and wires and set free for three or four hours. Mom would either take me home or to school to see my friends, or on occasion to the mall or the movies. Once I had to visit a hairdresser to have the vicious knots at the back of my head detangled after lying in bed so much. But every day by 5:00 P.M. I had to report back to the hospital to be tethered once again to that silver pole.

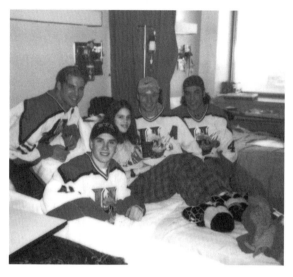

Members of the Halifax Mooseheads hockey team visited fifteen-year-old Heather at the IWK Health Centre in February 1998.

The hospital often had free tickets to the Halifax Mooseheads hockey games, the city's major junior team, where I would use my "free time" on occasion to go with my parents. It was there that I also met a friend—a girl named Julie, who was in the hospital at the same time as me for treatment of her Crohn's disease. Our parents got to talking, making the connection that we were all using hockey tickets from the hospital. It turned out we were just down the hall from one another, me in the east wing, her in the west. After that night, we connected

Total parenteral nutrition (TPN) is a method of feeding used to provide nutrition when a person can't eat. A formula is administered through a vein to bypass the gastrointestinal tract.

in the hospital a bit, hanging out in the teen lounge, where Mooseheads players would come to visit, much to our delight as fifteen-year-olds.

Along with the liquid nutrition pumping through my veins, medications were dripped into my body, including a nasty, evil (or so I thought) steroid called prednisone, used to help reduce inflammation. The drug made my face swell and puff up, leaving me with fat chipmunk cheeks. I cried when I looked in the mirror a few days after the first dose. It also caused aching pain in my joints, gave me difficulty sleeping, and created terrible mood swings. I hated the side effects but wasn't left with much choice—I'd have been much worse off without it.

Gradually, the treatment I was receiving in hospital started to pay off. I felt better and stronger as each day passed. Slowly, Dr. Ste-Marie let me eat again, starting with a piece of gum, then ice chips, then clear fluids. Finally, I was allowed to eat real food again, and for the first time in a long time, it didn't hurt. I was allowed to go home. The ulcerative colitis had gone into remission. Or so I hoped.

Being diagnosed with a chronic illness did have its silver lining. One afternoon my dad arrived at the hospital with exciting news. My parents had splurged and booked a trip to Florida for that spring. They'd be taking my niece (eight years younger than me) and me to Disney World and then to Coco Beach for a few days on the coast. My family had never taken a vacation like this before, and I was pleased as punch to be the beneficiary of this pick-me-up perk.

As time went on, the disease seemed to lurk, nagging at my insides, trying to break loose and rip through my intestines like a raging fire. But I was up for the battle. I'd been taking Asacol (mesalamine), a medication that reduces inflammation in the bowel—six pills a day from the day I was first diagnosed. But it wasn't enough on its own. The aches and pains and cramps kept returning.

One after the other, I tried the drugs commonly used to treat ulcerative colitis. The problem was, I had a bad reaction to most of them. One messed up my liver enzymes; one inflamed my pancreas, and another resulted in a blotchy, purple rash. I tried many of the 5-ASA (5-aminosalicylic acid) medications—Asacol, Salofalk, and Pentasa—drugs that reduce inflammation and allow damaged tissue to heal. I tried Losec (omeprazole), a proton pump inhibitor used to treat ulcers; azathioprine (Imuran), an immunosuppressive agent to calm the immune system and reduce irritation; hydrocortisone, a steroid that calms the body's immune response; Prevacid (lansoprazole), yet another proton pump inhibitor that heals ulcers; and ranitidine, a histamine blocker used to treat and prevent ulcers.

Prednisone was tried and true, although the doctors were reluctant to leave me on it for too long because of the long-term side effects: softening of the bones, reduced immunity, cataracts, and high blood pressure. Like a yo-yo, I went on and off that drug, sometimes taking sixteen pills a day. It was the only thing that worked; the only thing that could keep me going.

And so it went through my three years of high school. Along with the typical self-esteem and confidence issues most teenagers are faced with, I was fighting a constant battle against an unattractive disease that left my body wrecked from potent drugs and their ugly side effects. My face morphed from skeletal to chubby with each prescription of steroids, and I was always pale because of low iron in my blood. I'd lose weight as fast as I could gain it, my appetite constantly fluctuating—from non-existent when I was sick to ravenous when I was feeling good. I was self-conscious about my appearance at times but no one ever said a thing—at least not to my face. I was never teased or made to feel uncomfortable. I stayed out of the hospital, and I continued to live my life. I wasn't going to let the disease get in my way.

"Have you heard of a disease called ulcerative colitis?" I asked. Matt and I were sitting on the big white couch in his living room. It was a crisp October night in the fall of 2001, a few weeks after we'd met, and we were having one of those long, late-night conversations people sometimes have when they're getting to know one another. It was well after midnight, but we were still filling each other in on our very different lives. Matt, eighteen years old, had spent the previous eight years at a boarding school in England while his parents moved around the world. I was about to turn nineteen and I'd lived in the same suburban community of Bedford, just outside Halifax, for the past fourteen years. He was full of interesting stories from time spent in Japan, England, Malta, Bahrain, and Dubai. He seemed a little too good to be true—this athletic, well-travelled, cultured, and attractive guy with a sexy Scottish accent. We'd just started at the same university and had the same classes. There was something about the way our relationship was so comfortable from the start that I felt I could tell him about being sick. Friends I had grown up with knew about it because they'd been there as it happened, but it was the first time I'd spoken the words myself. As much as he'd seen and done around the world, he hadn't heard of this disease. I told him what it was, how I took medication for it every day, how I'd been sick before, how I might get sick again. I wasn't sure he quite understood what it all meant, but he was concerned. Most importantly, he said, "Okay, well, I'm here for you."

April 17, 2002

Dear Diary,

I couldn't have asked to meet a better person in my life. I just feel like he understands everything. He understands, and he cares. Being sick is almost easy having him around. I can handle this with his help.

Matt sat at the end of my hospital bed. He was all dressed up for his big night on the town—his nineteenth birthday. The top few buttons of his blue shirt were undone, revealing a white T-shirt underneath; his sleeves were rolled up to his elbows. He was wearing my favourite navy pants, and his hair was gelled just the way I liked it. I sat there in my pyjamas wearing no makeup, my hair a big mess. I hadn't even showered in days.

I couldn't celebrate with him. He promised me it was okay, but I could see the disappointment in his face. I was furious to be missing out. Finally, we were both of legal drinking age and I couldn't even take Matt out for a drink. He told me he was headed to the Wardroom, our college bar, and then probably to some local pubs. He'd dropped in to see me on his way out, so I gave him a hug and told him to have fun. He promised to come back the next day for a longer visit.

Later, as I lay wide awake in my bed, I heard the voices of young people whooping and hollering as they passed the building. Even up on the ninth floor I could hear them making their way home from the bars. Jealous, I wondered if Matt was among them.

I'd been in the hospital for a few days and had graduated from the IWK to the adult hospital—the Victoria General (VG), which is part of the QEII Health Sciences Centre. But I'd been sick for weeks. I'd missed tons of classes and spent most days dozing on the couch, feeling like I had some horrible flu. I had a constant fever, my mouth was full of canker sores, and a rash of red and purple bumps had developed on my legs—a condition called erythema nodosum, a common manifestation of Crohn's that can flare up along with intestinal inflammation. A few days earlier, the GI clinic had managed to squeeze me in for an emergency appointment with Dr. Munaa Khaliq-Kareemi, who would be my new gastroenterologist. He's a friendly, soft-spoken man who genuinely cares about his patients, letting them help determine their own treatment. He knew I hated prednisone, and he cared about helping me find a better alternative, although there really wasn't one. And I knew he knew best. When he saw the condition I was in, he wouldn't let me leave the hospital. Blood tests detected an infection in my blood. He wanted me on a heavy dose of steroids and antibiotics, and an IV would get them through my system faster than taking medication orally.

Dr. Kareemi was a little perplexed by my condition. The symptoms were looking more and more like those of Crohn's disease. Or maybe I had Crohn's colitis, a rare combination of the two. Either way, it was all the same to me. Change the diagnosis a hundred times over but it was still the same unfortunate enigmatic curse that I was stuck with.

After only a few days, I was itching to get out of the hospital. Final exams were looming, but more importantly so was the trip to Florida I'd been planning with my girlfriends to kick off the summer holidays. I did not intend to miss this trip. After only a week, I begged and pleaded with Dr. Kareemi to let me go home. I wasn't 100 percent healthy, but I promised him I was feeling a whole lot better. It may have been a bit of a lie, but I was feeling a little bit better.

Maybe I should have been a patient patient and stayed longer, waiting until I really felt back to normal. But that's part of the problem with people who have a chronic illness: they begin to think pain is normal. Perhaps that's why I spent that summer keeping only one small step ahead of a flare-up I knew was lingering inside, nagging at my insides, waiting to strike. I could feel it brewing.

Running on the power of steroids, I made it on the girls' trip to Florida. I had a great time, but with eyes on the nearest

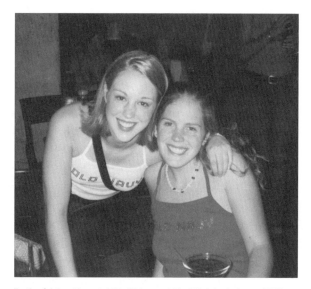

Heather (pictured here at right with her good friend Christina in August 2002) was good at hiding how unwell she was feeling, even during a flare-up of symptoms, which she was experiencing during this late-night birthday celebration for a friend.

bathroom at all times. By the end of the summer, I was experiencing a full-on flare-up. I'd stopped eating again, only nibbling here and there when I had the strength to endure the pain as the food progressed through my system.

"You're not going out," my mom told me, spotting me slumped over late one night near the end of August.

"Yeah, I am," I responded. I'd just gotten home from a six-hour shift at the gas station where I worked part-time. It was 11:30 P.M., my body ached, and I was exhausted, but I still went downstairs to my room, got changed, redid my makeup, and went upstairs to the kitchen. I sat down, resting my head on the table as I waited for my friends to pick me up.

It was Jenn's birthday and a bunch of us had bought matching halter tops when we were shopping in Florida. We all planned to wear them that night and I wasn't going to be the one to miss out. A car beeped in the driveway, and I dashed out the door, mustering all the energy I could from some unknown place inside. I faked being fine to make it through the night and managed to keep up with my friends. They were none the wiser that I was so unwell.

I also refused to miss out on the first week back at university. It was frosh week and my friends and I were all frosh leaders. Every day was a different activity, every night a different party. I pushed myself and pushed my body, participating in just about everything. The only night I cut short was after a hot day at the beach. I was sunburned and severely dehydrated; I had a smashing headache so intense it brought me to tears, my head pounding with every step I took. I had no choice but to go home and pass out in my bed.

My mom was not impressed, insisting each day that I cut it out, or at least stop drinking alcohol, which was probably the worst thing I could be doing to my already ravaged insides. My reasoning was that I was already sick, what would a little alcohol do? Besides, I knew the fun only lasted a week; I could rest as much as I wanted once it was over. But this time I pushed my body a little too far.

"Matt, I'm not going to make it," I said. I'd never felt so weak. We were walking across campus, and I had completely run out of steam. I couldn't go any farther; I dropped to the curb.

"Well, you can't just stay here," he said. At a loss, we both sat there on the ground; I was slumped in his arms.

I'd made it to the first three days of classes—the days where the professor hands out the syllabus and sends you on your way. On the third day, Matt and I had an evening class together: Psychology 1000. It lasted all of ten minutes, thankfully, but even then, I had to leave, running to the bathroom, sick to my stomach. Matt had soccer practice after class but wanted to walk me to my car first.

After a few moments on the ground, we finally decided Matt should go get my car and bring it to me. There was no way I could walk the rest of the way. He set off at a run, leaving me behind. By the time he got back, I felt like I could drive myself home. Assuring Matt I'd be all right, I set off for home and he headed to the field for practice.

I made it, barely, staggering through the front door and collapsing on the couch. For a change, Dad was in charge of supper—meatloaf. He brought a plate of it to me on the couch, and for some unknown reason I ate it. Devoured it. Every last crumb. I gulped down glasses of strawberry-banana juice. It was fantastic. It was also a huge mistake.

The night that followed was gruelling, the pain relentless. I woke up every ten minutes, dashing to the bathroom bent over in agony. I had crazy dreams in which I was attached to an IV pole that introduced itself as Mr. Denis Coderre, the minister of citizenship and immigration. He kept introducing himself over and over, in a thick French accent. Matt had just interviewed Coderre for a journalism assignment, but I had no idea why he was in my mind that night, of all nights. I knew nothing about the man, but after having his name run through my mind over and over that night, I can't say I was too fond of him. I was pretty sure I was losing my mind.

The next day was Friday the thirteenth: definitely not my lucky day. But at least the unbearable night had passed. Fortunately, I had an appointment to see Dr. Kareemi that morning. I waited for him in the examining room, sprawled out on the examining table, much too weak to sit up on my own. I'd lost weight again from not eating, and my organs were going to start shutting down if I didn't get some sort of nutrition into my body. It was time for more TPN, this time pumped in through a major vein in my arm, instead of my chest. It was also time for another round of intravenous steroids.

My oldest sister had brought me to this appointment, and I hadn't packed a bag to bring with me this time. I made a list of the things I needed, and she headed home to collect them for me while I waited for my room to be ready. As soon as I got there, I picked up the phone beside my bed and called Matt.

"How was your appointment?" he asked.

"They aren't letting me go home."

"Okay. I'm coming to see you." He knew where to find me—up on the ninth floor, once again. I didn't feel scared. I simply opened the *Harry Potter* book I had brought with me because I was conscious of the long waiting times to get in to see the doctor. Ignoring the three other patients sharing the room, I sat and read and didn't really feel anything, apart from feeling sick. Perhaps I was just used to the routine. I was there for some IV treatment. I'd done this before; I could do it again. Perhaps I would have felt differently if I'd known what was ahead.

There was no time to be bored in the hospital with a family like mine. I was rarely alone, except at night when it was time to sleep. I might be on my own for an hour or two some afternoons or evenings, but only when the rest of the family was assured there was something good on TV; my parents would never deny me the luxury of that grey, thirteen-inch fuzzy television screen that protruded from the wall on its long swivelling arm—even at the cost of fifteen dollars a day.

My mom was there first thing every morning, running water into a washbasin, and digging clothes out of my locker. It wasn't an easy task, trying to change clothes while attached to a pole. Every day Dad came by on his lunch break or after work. My older sisters and their families came in to play games; my older brother would drop by cracking jokes. It all made being in the hospital almost...fun.

I could see in Matt's eyes how tired he was when he came to visit. He had such a hectic schedule: he was back at school, working part-time, playing soccer—and he was the team's star at that. But he came every day. He helped me put my hair up, he read to me, and he even recorded his voice on tape so he could be there with me when he couldn't physically be there. He was always by my side.

On September 19, Matt arrived at the hospital with two purple roses—my favourite colour—in a pretty porcelain vase. The nurses all turned a blind eye as he marched past the "No flowers please" posters that lined the corridor, reminding visitors of the scent-free policy. The nurse assigned to my care that night knew it was our one-year anniversary and compassionately let me keep the flowers by my bed. Our romantic dinner consisted of Matt eating everything off my hospital dinner tray, and me eating two spoonfuls of soup. I wasn't feeling up to a trip to the common room next door, so Matt squished onto the bed beside me, setting up the laptop so we could watch one of the DVDs he'd rented. Keeping the volume low so as not to disturb the other patients, we strained to hear *The Royal Tenenbaums* as nurses bustled in and out, taking care of the other patients in the room. I didn't care what we were doing, I was just happy to be spending time with Matt.

The movie ended, and we turned our attention to my little TV. It was the season premiere of *Friends* that night, and a new season of *Survivor* was starting. Matt's dad wouldn't be picking him up until the shows were over at 11:00 P.M. By now the nurses were making the bedtime rounds, handing out meds and getting everyone settled in for the night. I heard the old woman in the bed across from me complaining to the nurse, insulted that Matt and I were sitting on the same bed, so close. She suggested that it was probably time for him to leave. My temper started to soar. I was not about to let this woman ruin my night, and thankfully, neither was the nurse. As long as we were keeping quiet—as we had the whole evening—she saw nothing wrong with what we were doing. Matt was allowed to stay and visit as late as he wanted.

The treatment I was receiving in the hospital wasn't working. I had been there nearly two weeks and I was only getting worse. I didn't even have to actually eat now to have the sharp, stabbing pains rip across my abdomen. One day a cupcake came with my lunch tray—a beautiful white cupcake with vanilla icing. (It may have been a trick to get me to eat something.) I touched nothing on the tray, but I saved that cupcake, waiting for the perfect moment. Later, when I decided I'd been looking at it for far too long, I couldn't resist. I took a tiny bite. The cake barely touched my tongue when my stomach muscles clenched, and it felt like my insides were twisting and turning, warning me not to eat any more.

The doctors decided the intravenous steroids weren't working anymore. A person could only depend on TPN for so long. The flare-up was out of control, too severe to tame into remission this way.

It was September 2002. Dr. Kareemi was out of town, but Dr. Desmond Leddin, the head of the division of digestive care and endoscopy, had taken over my case. He decided it was time to sit down and discuss the situation.

I had been dreading the meeting. Usually, the doctors just pulled the curtain around my hospital bed to create some "privacy" when they wanted to talk. But this time, I'd shuffled up the hallway of the hospital, making my way up to the conference room, so tired and weak I could barely stand. The short walk from my room felt like miles, but I refused to use a wheelchair. I could walk on my own. My mom had to push the IV pole, weighed down as it was with its monitors and bags of liquid dripping into the central line that was inserted in the major vein of my arm. I had no strength to push.

The thought running through my mind as I made my way up the hall was that this conference room was where doctors gathered families to deliver bad news, or where patients were faced with crucial decisions. I was only nineteen years old and felt it was truly unfair that I was in this situation. The fact that all these busy doctors were making time to sit down in a meeting with me was frightening. I had a feeling I was not going to want to hear what they had to say.

Leafy green plants decorated the conference room, accenting the stark white walls. A grey oval table sat in the middle of the room. There wasn't much more to it. Taking a seat at the table, my mom beside me and my dad beside her, I left several empty chairs to distance myself from Dr. Leddin—a tall, broad man with an authoritative aura, but who was really just a big teddy bear. He sat at the head of the table. A panel of professionals sat across from us: Dr. Stacey Williams, the young resident gastroenterologist, Dr. Christopher Jamieson, a talented surgeon, and two other men I was not familiar with in white lab coats. I felt small and timid facing these doctors, waiting for them to lay it all out.

Something, they said, had to be done because I wasn't getting any better. In fact, I was only getting worse.

This is one of the worst cases we've seen in a while...

Your gut is ripped apart...

Hardly any tissue left...

Tiny ulcers have exploded throughout the intestines...

The doctors' comments bombarded me. On a scale of one to ten, with ten being the worst, they'd given me an eight. I was in horrible condition with few options. They told me I could try yet more medication—this time, a new experimental drug called Remicade. The known side effects are like those from chemotherapy. Other side effects? They didn't know. It would be a long process, with more hospitalizations as the drug destroyed my immune system. They didn't even know if it would help.

Or...I could have surgery, a major surgery. They could remove the diseased part of my insides and then—maybe—I could have my life back. My parents asked question after question, but I just sat there, stone-faced, listening to what was being said. Once they all finished talking, the room was quiet. It was my turn; everyone faced me, anticipating what I might say. They wanted to know what I was thinking. I was silent.

Finally, Dr. Leddin spoke. He told me I had a very good poker face—the best he had ever seen.

When they were finished, I left the conference room and shuffled back down the hallway to my room, still silent, my mom pushing the IV pole for me once again. I didn't know what to think. I didn't know what to say. I didn't know what to do. We crept along in silence, past the kitchen on the right, the nurses' station on the left, and finally into room 91A, where I collapsed onto my bed, into my boyfriend's arms, and burst into tears.

I had a daunting decision to make, and I was the only one who could make it. It didn't matter what anyone else thought; ultimately the choice was mine. At least I knew that no matter what I decided—whether it was rounds of experimental medication and more hospitalizations, or a major surgery that would leave my intestine hanging out of a hole in my side—I'd have a lot of support.

As frightened and confused as I felt, I began to realize that, deep down, I knew what really had to be done. I remembered

Normal Anatomy

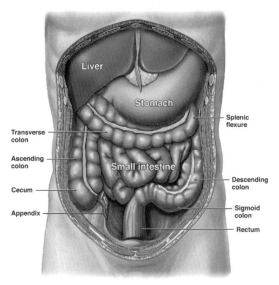

Liver

Stomach

Splenic flexure

Transverse colon

Ascending colon

Cecum

Appendix

Small intestine

Descending colon

Sigmoid colon

Rectum

Anterior view

Post-colectomy

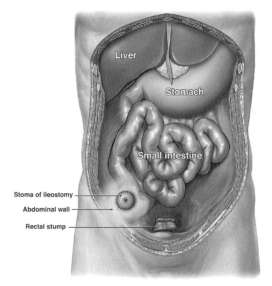

Liver

Stomach

Small intestine

Stoma of ileostomy

Abdominal wall

Rectal stump

An illustration of a complete colectomy (colon removal) with ileostomy surgery. Pictured at top, a typical digestive system. The post-operative diagram, left, shows that the large colon has been removed and a small portion of the small intestine has been passed through the abdominal wall to create an ileostomy stoma.

back to that very first day in Dr. Ste-Marie's office, at the beginning of this whole tumultuous experience. She had advised me that if I ever needed surgery, my body would let me know when it was time. I had been in pain for so long the prospect of relief was exciting. I was sick and tired of being sick and tired. I wanted to go home. I wanted to go back to university. I wanted my life back. It was time.

The surgery took place three days after my decision. I had a subtotal colectomy, in which the surgeon removed the diseased colon, saving about five centimetres of my sigmoid colon. My ileum, the lower part of my small intestine, was connected to an opening in my abdomen, called a stoma or ostomy, that was covered with a pouch to collect what normally passes through the digestive tract. One reason I was willing to subject myself to this awkward new lifestyle was knowing I could have a second surgery in six months, once I healed, to reconnect everything inside. Still, the lingering thought in the back of my mind was that the disease could come back full force, any day, any time.

Waking up in the recovery room was a terrifying moment. I could hear nurses calling my name from far away, but I couldn't breathe, move, or see. Eventually I came to and realized immediately I was feeling no pain. Of course, I was hopped up on painkillers—strong drugs were running through my blood, and I'd had an epidural that had frozen my abdomen so I couldn't feel a thing. But it was blissful. They'd wheeled me into the operating room (OR) at noon; by 10:00 P.M. that night I was sitting up in bed, chatting away with my parents. I was just out of surgery and felt better than I could remember for a long time.

October 8, 2002

Dear Diary,

Coming home was one of the best feelings in my life. I felt so unbelievably good! For once, I'm going to be healthy. I can go out and enjoy everything that I do. It hasn't even been two weeks since my surgery. I'm only beginning this new…what would you call it, journey? Adventure? Life? But the hell I went through is over. I pray I stay healthy. I've learned a lot about life, about myself, about other people. I just can't believe I've been through so much. I'm not sure why either, but I am sure I now appreciate life so much more.

THE LONG AND WINDING ROAD TO DIAGNOSIS

The journey to diagnosis can be the hardest part of having IBD, says Barbara Currie, who has over sixteen years of experience as an IBD nurse practitioner with the Nova Scotia Collaborative IBD Program and the division of digestive care and endoscopy at the QEII Health Sciences Centre. Many patients will wait years for a diagnosis of IBD but it can happen more quickly if they end up in hospital with severe symptoms.

For those with mild to moderate symptoms, the journey to diagnosis can be very challenging. "They have these symptoms, they go for blood work, and the blood work doesn't show a whole lot," says Currie. "And particularly in the last few years [since Covid-19], with diagnostic imaging being more challenging to access, getting scans and seeing evidence of more small bowel involvement is tricky."

Getting a referral to gastroenterology can be delayed in the absence of alarming symptoms like rectal bleeding, significant weight loss, and severe changes in blood work. "Wait times are long to see a gastroenterologist for a confirmation of a diagnosis of IBD," explains Currie. Once a patient gets a diagnosis, the path forward should become clearer—if still scary.

"They've likely had a colonoscopy or some diagnostic imaging [and] more advanced blood work," says Currie. "We then have a sense of yes, this is IBD, this is Crohn's or ulcerative colitis or a variation of either, like an indeterminate colitis, and here's the severity and here are our treatment options." She says that while it's not the kind of news anyone particularly wants to hear, at least they're finally getting some answers. A course can then be outlined, plans can be defined, and directions determined for which route to take, depending on how the patient wants to get to remission.

A FORK IN THE ROAD

But even along the journey to a diagnosis of IBD, there is a different route to discovering Crohn's disease than ulcerative colitis. One is more like a direct route straight up the highway and the other takes a winding road.

"Crohn's can be more insidious and a little bit more difficult to get to the diagnosis unless it's an urgent presentation," says Currie. She describes the potential path for each.

With Crohn's disease, a patient can feel unwell for years. They may have bloating, abdominal pain, and fluctuations in their bowel habits. Sometimes these are so bad the patient restricts their diet. Their blood work might not be too bad; they may be referred to gastroenterology for a colonoscopy, but there's no evidence of disease. They may be told they have Irritable Bowel Syndrome (or IBS, a separate and distinct gastrointestinal disorder that affects the gastrointestinal tract with similar symptoms, while IBD involves the inflammation or chronic swelling of the intestines). The patient may trek along thinking they have IBS, but things get worse. Blood work starts showing some alterations. White blood cell counts go up; hemoglobin goes down; inflammatory markers are elevating; iron stores are lowering. Now there's evidence that there's active inflammation present that would not be seen with IBS. The patient is referred again to gastroenterology, and this time they get a scope.

"The nice thing now is we do have the ability for primary care providers to connect with GI on a quick consult basis," says Currie. "We could at that time arrange for a stool specimen for calprotectin, which we now have as a non-invasive, easy test that acts as a surrogate marker of disease activity."

The laboratory test screens for calprotectin, a protein that is detected when some part of the body is inflamed. Stool infections and C. difficile (a bacterial infection) can also be ruled out by the primary care provider ordering stool culture and sensitivity testing to make sure there isn't anything compounding the patient's symptoms.

"If the stool cultures are negative and the fecal calprotectin is quite elevated, we have a pretty good sense that this person likely has inflammatory bowel disease," says Currie. "We don't know exactly where it is yet, and we don't know if it's Crohn's or ulcerative colitis, but we know that there's inflammation in the gastrointestinal tract and further investigation is warranted. So that's often what a Crohn's patient's journey looks like."

For ulcerative colitis, Currie explains a diagnosis can be arrived at a little bit more quickly because people with ulcerative colitis often present with rectal bleeding, which is always an alarm signal. "You get action a whole lot quicker when you're bleeding rectally," says Currie. "And often they're

A scope (or endoscopic examination) is a procedure to check for signs of inflammation in the GI tract. The main types of endoscopic testing are upper endoscopy and colonoscopy. An endoscopy is a procedure in which an endoscope—a flexible tube with a small camera and light on one end— is fed through the mouth to look inside the upper gut (esophagus, stomach) and small intestine. A colonoscopy (also referred to as a sigmoidoscopy) is a procedure in which a sigmoidoscope, or scope—a narrow, flexible tube with a light and a tiny camera on one end—is passed through the rectum all the way through the large intestine and into the last part of the small intestine to check for areas of inflammation or lesions.

having significant diarrhea, they often have more rapid weight loss, they have more alterations in their blood work sooner because when the large bowel gets sick, the patient is very sick."

Because ulcerative colitis starts in the rectum, the patient is often very symptomatic with feelings of urgency and incomplete emptying, says Currie. They may not be able to go to work or school, they're up all through the night with bowel movements, and they feel absolutely miserable. These patients may show up in the emergency department because rectal bleeding is alarming. They're often anemic and have very low albumin, a protein made by the liver. Inflammatory markers are often quite high, and they'll often present and be scoped on a more urgent basis. Because evidence of ulcerative colitis is more obvious, treatment is sometimes initiated sooner.

The ileocecal region is a portion of the digestive tract that comprises the cecum (a pouch that forms the first part of the large intestine; it connects the small intestine to the colon), the appendix, the terminal ileum (the last and longest section of the small intestine), and the ileocecal valve (a sphincter muscle at the junction of the ileum and the colon that allows digested food to pass from the small intestine into the large intestine).

"Sometimes things are so severe a patient requires hospitalization with ulcerative colitis—if it's an acute, severe presentation," says Currie. With Crohn's, the evidence is not always as obvious, unless the patient has a bowel obstruction.

"If somebody has severe right lower quadrant abdominal pain and they're suspicious of appendicitis so they go to the [emergency room], that can be an acute presentation or sudden presentation with Crohn's," says Currie.

A bowel obstruction may

occur because a patient has long-standing scar tissue right where the small bowel meets the large bowel and the ileocecal region. Because Crohn's is a disease that can involve all layers of the bowel, there can be scarring. The patient will eventually—and urgently—experience a bowel obstruction. They can also develop abscesses or fistulas that work their way outside the bowel, leading to infection and perforations. These are more acute presentations of Crohn's, but they certainly happen.

A fistula is a small tunnel that can form through parts of the intestine. It can connect to other sections of intestine, to the skin, or to other internal organs. Sometimes fistulas can burrow to the skin or to a blind end where fluid can accumulate. If the fluid becomes infected, it is called an abscess.

– *Source: Crohn's and Colitis Canada*

THE CHALLENGE OF TREATMENT

Once a patient has a diagnosis, the conversations around treatment and medication management can also be quite difficult.

"In my experience over many years, the treatment journey is sometimes a difficult one because the language of treatment options can be terrifying to patients," says Currie. "We're talking about biologic therapy [a type of disease treatment that uses substances made from living organisms], we're talking about all the potential side effects of biologic therapy and immunosuppressant therapy, and what's not always being said to the patient…is—'What are the risks of not doing anything?'"

Biologic therapies can be very effective at settling down the disease. Biologic drugs are made from living cells and they act as immunosuppressants to help stop inflammation in the body. Inflammation can be a good thing, helping your immune system fight a possible threat. An overactive immune system may damage healthy tissue. The use of biologic therapies can block inflammation in the gut, allowing the disease to heal inside.

Biologics are powerful drugs, though, and their use raises the risk of infection due to suppression of the immune system; it can also cause rare tumour growth and can slightly raise the risk of developing certain types of skin cancer. Allergic reactions are also possible. But Currie says the risk of doing nothing— or not escalating to the best therapy options available—is far riskier than the treatments themselves or any of the potential side effects of the treatments.

"We don't talk about that enough in the mainstay conversation," says Currie. "So I make a note of always talking about options. We typically have three options: you can do nothing, which is probably never a very good option; we can start with this or that medication; or we can sometimes lead with the most effective medicines that we have today to treat inflammatory bowel disease, which at the end of the day are biologics."

Currie compares the advancements in the use of biologic therapy in IBD to its use in the context of other health issues.

"If we look at the advancements in cancer therapies over the last ten years specifically, they've all moved to almost all biologic, targeted therapies. Why? Because they're the best. And sometimes people forget, or maybe they just don't know that we have these advanced therapies for the treatment of IBD. We're so fortunate to have them."

The greatest challenge for practitioners is the inability to accurately predict whether a particular therapy is going to work for a specific patient.

"That's where the advancements in the future will help us," says Currie. "And that's a difficult journey for patients.

They put their trust in the clinician to recommend the best, safest, most effective treatment. And then sometimes they have a partial response, or a loss of response over time. And that is discouraging. It's discouraging for the clinician too, because we hope that it's going to be the best treatment for our patient. But we don't have the ability to genotype a patient and say, 'Medications A, B, and C are not going to work for you, but medications D, E, and F will, so we're going to start with medication D.' …We're not there yet. Someday we might be there, and that will help the patient's journey tremendously because we'll likely be able to induce remission faster." Currie says that, at the end of the day, all the biologics probably have similar efficacy in IBD.

"The best-case scenario is [that] 30 to 40 percent of patients who are treated with a biologic have meaningful, sustained clinical remission. We always run the risk of patients losing response or developing antibodies to our current biologics, which are fairly large proteins. And because they're proteins, the body's pretty smart and says, 'Oh, look, there's a foreign protein in my bloodstream. I'm going to produce an antibody against that protein because it's not supposed to be here.' Some medications cause more immunogenicity, and the immunogenicity just means that the body produces antibodies to a particular drug. So in the future, we're looking at more small molecules that are oral and don't have any immunogenicity."

Currie suspects that future drugs now in development will recognize and identify pathways of inflammation that weren't fully understood even five years ago.

"That's very encouraging for people with immune [system] diseases and inflammatory diseases, because I think we're just going to get better and better at targeting the right pathway for a given patient, and with safer medications," she says. "The medications we use now are safe, but things can always be safer." Currie says she feels very fortunate to have seen the evolution of treatment options for patients. "I've seen how they've changed people's lives. They've reduced the need for surgeries. But they're not without their own challenges."

There are other components of the patient's journey that can be complex and stressful, like when moving off a parent's health insurance plan, entering the workforce and navigating insurance coverage, not having a drug plan, or retiring and moving to a provincial drug plan, which may have some limitations in terms of coverage.

Any way you look at it, medications are expensive, and Currie says without coverage patients can be left with less-than-optimal treatment choices. "Not so much in the biologic realm, because our pharma partners have been very gracious in providing compassionate drugs to patients," says Currie. "I have never had a patient in all my years go without biologic therapy in the absence of a drug plan."

LIFE WITH IBD

After the journey to diagnosis, then navigating treatment options and medication management, comes all the follow-up required to live with a chronic disease—a lifetime commitment to learning how to manage flare-ups (from minor to more serious), staying on top of medications and prescriptions, attending appointments and having tests done, knowing how to take care of yourself, and learning where to turn for help.

On top of all that, there's the stigma around talking about IBD. It's certainly not typical dinner conversation. People tend not to talk about it, or they only talk about it with certain people, or only with their health professionals. Living with IBD can be an isolating and lonely experience.

But as Currie says, there is hope. Crohn's and colitis are lifelong chronic conditions but can go into remission for years and years. Currie says she has seen the treatment of IBD come a long way in her years with the IBD clinic.

"I've seen the advancement of therapeutic treatment options explode in the last ten years; even in the last five years different targeted pathways of inflammation [have been] identified, with new treatments," she says. "I've seen significant improvements in patients' quality of life, and their time to remission. It's been wonderful in that way. We've been able to move away from steroids as the backbone of our treatment algorithm…to more complex proteins and biologics that are game changers in inflammatory bowel disease. Just seeing that progression has been awesome."

THE NOVA SCOTIA COLLABORATIVE IBD TEAM

D r. Jennifer Jones, team lead of the Nova Scotia Collaborative Inflammatory Bowel Diseases (NSCIBD) program, was born and raised in Cape Breton, NS. She decided at an early age she wanted to be a physician to help people—so she set out to do just that.

Jones obtained her medical degree and completed her internal medicine and gastroenterology fellowship training at Dalhousie University. When she worked with people living with IBD, she decided it was the field she wanted to focus on. She went on to complete an advanced clinical and research fellowship in inflammatory bowel diseases at the Mayo Clinic in Rochester, MN.

After moving to Calgary, AB, Jones worked in the IBD program at the University of Calgary, completing more training and research and earning an MSc in Epidemiology. She then moved to Saskatoon, SK, where she was able to put her knowledge into action.

"I was able, with the team, to build one of the first IBD programs that was multidisciplinary in nature," says Jones. She worked as an assistant professor of medicine at the University of Saskatchewan and established the first provincial multidisciplinary Inflammatory Bowel Diseases program at the Royal University Hospital in the Saskatchewan Health Region. After six years in Saskatoon, Jones made the move to Nova Scotia.

"This is my home," says Jones. "Family is here, loved ones are here. I viewed it as a privilege and an honour to be able to come back to a place that has so much IBD [where I could] use my skills and what I've learned to hopefully improve things for people living with IBD."

She's right about the need. In 2018, nearly 12,000 Nova Scotians had IBD. Jones is now the medical co-lead (along with colleague Dr. Michael Stewart) of the NSCIBD program and director of research for Dalhousie Medical School's division of digestive care and endoscopy; she also provides clinical care at the QEII Health Sciences Centre.

"I did additional training in implementation science so I would have the tools to be able to…change the health system to make improvements," she says. She's currently Director of Clinical Systems Innovation with the department of medicine as well.

Jones's dissatisfaction with patients' access to care—an issue she has observed everywhere in the country but perceives to be significantly worse in Nova Scotia—prompted her to help find a solution. The NSCIBD program is a group of practitioners, allied healthcare providers (including researchers, dieticians, and psychologists), and nursing specialists (consisting of nurse practitioners and a nurse navigator), as well as IBD-focussed gastroenterologists, whose collective goal is to improve the lives of people living with IBD in Nova Scotia.

"Our mission ultimately is to overcome barriers to access to multidisciplinary IBD care," says Jones. "When I moved back, the [division] already had two nurse practitioners, which was amazing. They were recruited and onboarded way back in the early 2000s when there was a big exodus of gastroenterologists. We were very fortunate that they were hired and stepped in to fill that care gap, which was absolutely critical."

The nurse practitioners with the NSCIBD program are Kelly Phalen-Kelly and Barbara Currie. Phalen-Kelly was the first IBD nurse practitioner in the country, joining the clinic in 2001. She was joined by Currie in 2006.

Barbara Currie has been in nursing for over thirty-five years. After finishing her baccalaureate in nursing at Dalhousie she went on to work in intensive care for ten years, then on to different areas, diabetes management among them. Currie pursued a master's degree in nursing in the nurse practitioner stream at the Dalhousie School of Nursing and in 2006 came to work with the division of gastroenterology (now the division of digestive care and endoscopy) as the third nurse practitioner specializing in IBD in the country.

Seventeen years later, they are both still there. Currie says the easiest way to describe a nurse practitioner's role is to imagine the role of nursing, then imagine the role of medicine, and bridge the two.

"At the end of the day, I'm always a nurse," says Currie. "I'm a registered nurse first, I'm a nurse practitioner second." With her nurse-practitioner education, Currie's scope of practice is expanded to include the ability to diagnose, manage, and treat illness, prescribe medicines, order diagnostic tests, monitor those tests, and consult with other clinicians as appropriate. "I have advanced knowledge and skill in inflammatory bowel disease. All I do all day long is inflammatory bowel disease— every day, all day. I develop an expertise, sometimes even more uniquely than, say, a community gastroenterologist who would see *all* things GI."

Currie explains how even within their own division, some gastroenterologists will refer a patient to Phalen-Kelly or to her for a second opinion on treatment or assessment because it is what they deal with every day, but she acknowledges she is not a medical doctor.

"I have not completed four years of internal medicine and a residency in gastroenterology. I certainly recognize that the contributions that medicine and nursing make are complementary and collaborative," she says, noting that about 20 percent of her work involves collaborating with a gastroenterologist "to manage the parts of that patient's inflammatory bowel disease that are more advanced or beyond my scope."

Situations beyond her scope could include a patient who needs to have dual biologic therapy (a treatment requiring two biologics), or who may have additional health problems that complicate their treatment course.

Along with a team of gastroenterologists and surgeons, the multidisciplinary team includes researchers, a dietitian, a clinical health psychologist, and a social worker when needed.

"Having a chronic illness does place some patients in a very marginalized group," says Currie. "Drug access can be expensive, and it can be stressful navigating insurance coverage." (See "Navigating Drug Coverage," page 53.)

Jones says that when she stepped into the group some clinical and educational resources existed. "What we've done since then is try to identify and build out those aspects of the program that we think need improvement, and [we] are still working on that."

One of the roles that's been added is a nurse navigator, a position Jones had seen in the Saskatoon program, which had been tremendously beneficial for patients and for the team.

"We provide support line access to our patients," says Currie. "That was one of the first things implemented when Kelly came into the role way back in 2001.... Because this is a chronic relapsing-remitting disease, patients need the ability to contact us when they're not well. We have a twenty-four-hour, seven day-a-week, 365-days-a year message centre where patients can call us, let us know the urgency of their call, and we do our best to get back to them if it's urgent within the twenty-four hours."

Previously, the nurse practitioners had been managing the patient support phone line, which Jones says took away from their ability to spend time with patients in the clinic. It reduced the overall number of people they could see and help.

The nurse navigator—Jessica Robar, a registered nurse—helps triage those calls and do further assessments to move the conversations along to the appropriate clinician. "The nurse navigator role is really that touchpoint between patients and the care team," says Jones. "The functions that Jess fills include anything from just answering a simple question about their disease or medications to fielding calls from individuals who are having flares of their disease. [It's about] getting investigations started and connecting with us about next steps."

The nurse practitioners play a big role in their patients' transition from pediatric care to adult care. They follow patients very closely as they begin to take on more responsibility for their own care. Currie adds that one of the big parts of her job is system navigation. "More recently, system navigation has become more and more complex, and people just don't know who to call. There's been a breakdown in primary care in this province. We know that many of our patients have no primary care providers [family doctors], so connecting patients with appropriate, basic health resources is a big part of our role." Currie describes her role as an all-inclusive position that runs the gamut of full nursing care to medical management.

"We do a lot of work with the patients around access to treatment, helping the patient better understand their diagnosis, their journey, and what to expect," says Currie. "This is a lifelong chronic disease…and our goal is that [patients] live the same life they would live without their Crohn's or their ulcerative colitis."

The NSCIBD program is not without its challenges. "There's a never-ending list of things to do," says Currie. "I think we need more nurses in the care of patients with inflammatory bowel disease not only as support people, but as frontline, first clinical contact. We need more training in inflammatory bowel disease for nurses because they will make a difference in access to care and time to treatment. Because waitlists for gastroenterologists are very long."

The NSCIBD program sees patients from all over the province, from Yarmouth to Cape Breton and everywhere in between, as well as patients from Prince Edward Island and New Brunswick on occasion.

"It's very rewarding," Currie says. "We have a wonderful team."

RESOURCES IN OTHER PROVINCES

QUEBEC

"The McGill IBD Research Group was established in 1992, by concerned members of the Montreal community who were affected by IBD, to ensure financial support for IBD clinics at the McGill University teaching hospitals. The group raises funds with the mandate to provide expert medical care, services, research, and resources to those living with IBD as well as their families."

Source: mcgillibd.ca

ONTARIO

"The IBD Centre at the Children's Hospital of Eastern Ontario (CHEO) in Ottawa provides a comprehensive multidisciplinary team approach to treatment of children diagnosed with IBD, striving to make a difference in the overall wellness of each child and youth."

Source: cheo.on.ca/en/clinics-services-programs/
inflammatory-bowel-disease-centre.aspx

"The IBD Clinic has been in place at the McMaster University Medical Centre (MUMC) of Hamilton Health Sciences since 2009 to provide patient-centred care for IBD patients. The IBD Clinic works as a multidisciplinary team and includes an advanced practice nurse, nutritionist, social worker, surgeons, and gastroenterologists to support patients with complicated or severe IBD."

Source: mcmasteribd.com

"Sinai Health's Centre for IBD, located at Mount Sinai Hospital in Toronto, is renowned for delivering excellence in patient care, education, and innovative research, advancing what's possible in the specialized care provided to patients living with IBD."

Source: mountsinai.on.ca/care/
inflammatory-bowel-disease

"The IBD Centre at SickKids Hospital in Toronto combines the expertise of SickKids' IBD program and the Research Institute to build on the understanding of the development of pediatric IBD, leading to better clinical care for pediatric patients. The SickKids IBD Centre exists to optimize the health and lives of children and youth with IBD and their families locally and globally."

Source: sickkids.ca/en/care-services/centres/
inflammatory-bowel-disease-centre

MANITOBA

"The IBD Clinical and Research Centre is a Manitoba-based network of clinicians, researchers, and trainees working collaboratively to improve health outcomes for people living with Crohn's disease and ulcerative colitis. The centre, which has received international attention and recognition for its research, has established among the largest IBD population databases in North America."

Source: ibdmanitoba.org

SASKATCHEWAN

"The Multidisciplinary IBD Clinic at the Royal University Hospital in the Saskatchewan Health Region provides patients with an interdisciplinary team of healthcare professionals who will assist them with the multifaceted management of their disease in order to control symptoms and prevent complications through in-depth educational sessions, support for administration of medications, and medical liaison."

Source: saskatoonhealthregion.ca/locations_services/Services/
cdm/Pages/Programs/Inflammatory-Bowel-Disease.aspx

ALBERTA

"The University of Alberta IBD Clinic provides world-class diagnosis and long-term treatment care for patients with IBD. The IBD Clinic is part of the parent organization IBD Unit, which encompasses academic and educational facilities bridging together research, education, and practice. The IBD Clinic sees individuals from northwestern Saskatchewan, eastern British Columbia, and the northern Territories."

Source: ibdclinic.ca

"The University of Calgary IBD Clinic is a multidisciplinary clinic dedicated to providing world-class care to patients diagnosed with IBD. They strive for excellence in the three key areas of patient care, clinical research, and patient/physician education."

Source: cumming.ucalgary.ca/departments/
medicine/divisionssections/gastroenterology/clinical/
inflammatory-bowel-disease-group

BRITISH COLUMBIA

"The IBD Centre of BC is committed to helping patients to develop a healthier and fulfilling life. The Centre's multidisciplinary teams draw upon a wide range of IBD-trained specialists to implement integrated, proactive, and personalized care based on patients' specific needs. Their goals are to deliver timely and efficient urgent care and proactive, ongoing health maintenance."

Source: ibdcentrebc.ca

MY STORY:
LIVING WITH AN
ILEOSTOMY (2002)

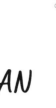

M y life-changing colectomy surgery on September 27, 2002, took not even two hours but it was followed by a long time in the recovery room. I had twenty staples holding my abdomen together, no more colon, and a bag stuck on my side where my intestine, my stoma, peeked out. My ileostomy. It was surprisingly easy to adjust to in those first days, largely because I was on a lot of pain medication, was elated to be healthy, and had so much support from my family and friends.

While I had welcomed the surgery—it dramatically improved my life—I was in no way adequately prepared for it. Back then, there was no social media. Google wasn't a popular verb. I don't recall ever even looking on the internet for information. When I was first diagnosed, my parents had bought a book called *Crohn's Disease and Ulcerative Colitis: Everything You Need To Know* by Fred Saibil, MD. It was our bible for all things Crohn's disease, a medical book filled with concise definitions, detailed tables, and diagrams—almost like an encyclopedia for IBD. A comprehensive review of the disease; accessible, but not very *personal*. Perhaps this was a blessing. In hindsight, I think the lack of information made the decision simpler. To be honest, if I'd known more at the impressionable age of nineteen about the physical outcome of the surgery, I might not have surrendered myself so quickly or confidently. But maybe there's just no amount of research in the world that will truly prepare you for what it's like to wake up with a surgically created opening in your abdomen that allows waste to leave your body. I didn't understand what I was in for until I was living it.

The hospital had a volunteer program where an experienced Crohnie would meet with a less experienced patient to talk about the disease you had in common. I remember being told there was one female volunteer under the age of seventy-five who'd had the same surgery, so of course that's who they set me up with. She came to see me in hospital during the days after my surgery. She was a successful business owner, and it was inspiring to meet a strong, independent woman who'd had the same experience as mine. It left a big impression; I vividly remember her walking in and sitting at my bedside. She was wearing tall boots with tights, a jean skirt, and a chic sweater. Phew. She looked totally normal, and I couldn't tell she had anything on the side of her belly. I don't remember much of the conversation, but I know it was mostly polite small talk. She told me the story of how she had been so sick she'd begged her doctors for her surgery—and had never looked back. That helped me feel good about the decision I'd made.

I was grateful I had even a little time to process the decision, unlike one of my hospital roommates, not much older than me, who had cycled in and out of the hospital and woke up one day with an ostomy after an emergency surgery for a bowel perforation. She was soon transferred to another room and I never saw her again. But even with some time to process, I was naive when I went into the surgery.

Days before the surgery I was provided with a pamphlet titled *Living With Your Ileostomy: A Guide to Self-Care*. Inside, there was an illustration of a post-surgery patient with a cute little red button on their side. No big deal at all. Yet when I looked down post-surgery, days later—nurses took care of everything going on down there for the first few days—I was absolutely shocked. It looked like a tongue was sticking out through the side of my stomach. A fat red tongue, with little bumpy taste buds pulsating out of my gut. Like a scene straight out of a horror film like *Alien* (an interesting fact is that screenwriter Dan O'Bannon actually credited his experiences with Crohn's disease for inspiring the infamous chest-bursting scene from the film). I couldn't believe part of my body, a part that was supposed to be on the inside, was poking outside of me and everyone at the hospital was just cool with it. But it was too late to turn back. I was feeling euphoric to be relieved of my symptoms. And besides, it was temporary. I steeled myself with the notion that this was a short-term, makeshift solution to fix all the sickness I'd endured. I couldn't decide whether I was upset or not that the medical team hadn't done more to prepare me for the reality of a stoma. Would it have really been helpful?

Recovery from the surgery turned out to be a little more challenging than I had imagined. Days after the surgery, my best friend, Christina, who I'd been close with since junior high school (pre-diagnosis), had come to the city for a visit. She'd agreed to take on the task of straightening my hair for me. My thick curls were in quite a state after so much time in the hospital, but I'd finally had the strength to wash it for the first time since the surgery. I thought I'd feel good with a nice, stylish blowout and then I wouldn't have to worry about my hair again until I was home.

Christina had helped me shuffle down the hall to the family room—a much different shuffle than the one I'd taken not too many days before with my parents on the way to the conference room. I pushed my own IV pole for support, my other hand gently clutching my stapled-up abdomen. I felt like I had to physically hold my belly together with every timid step forward.

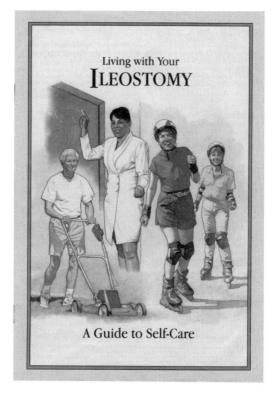

Living with Your
ILEOSTOMY

A Guide to Self-Care

Heather was presented with this pamphlet, titled *Living With Your Ileostomy: A Guide to Self-Care*, a few days before her surgery. It played down the physical manifestations of the surgery.

We sat in the family lounge, chatting away; I was having a good time for the first time in quite a while. Suddenly the dry hospital air caught in the back of my throat, and I started coughing. Coughing with a massive incision in my abdomen was agonizing. Between coughs I was groaning in pain and couldn't catch my breath.

Christina helped me stumble back up the hallway, where we ran into my nurse.

"Let's get you back to bed," the nurse directed, then gave me extra pain meds. Just like that, the meds made me drowsy and our "girl time" was over. Christina headed out as I nodded off, half of my hair straightened, half a rat's nest atop my head.

More friends came to visit to help cheer me up while I recovered in hospital, telling funny stories that made me laugh until it hurt—literally. Over time, I told my friends I'd had surgery to help my Crohn's disease, revealing I had some transitions to make as I embarked on a healthier life, but shared none of the gory details. I also remember sending an email from my Hotmail account to other friends about the surgery. Matt told me he was proud of me for sharing the information, yet I still kept the really personal stuff private. A few of my closest friends knew about the ostomy; I can't remember whether Matt told them or I did.

My ileostomy also remained physically hidden as well. A few people asked to see the bag and I'd show them the opaque plastic pouch attached to my stomach. But I did not show the stoma, which I called Stanley (how original), to a single soul; only my mother saw it. She had to help me with bag changes in the beginning until I got used to managing it on my own. While I had to empty out the contents of the bag a few times daily, every few days I had to peel the sticky connecting appliance off my skin, toss it out, and apply a new one. I remember standing in front of the mirror of the bathroom—the bathroom I'd spent so many sleepless nights rushing into with vomiting and diarrhea—with supplies spread across the vanity in front of me as I cut out flanges and sticky clay to stick the bag to my skin. It felt methodical and very businesslike. No sentiment attached. No one else ever saw the red pulsating stoma tongue—not even Matt.

I worried about my shirt riding up and revealing the bag, so my mom set my grandmother to work crafting cute fabric covers for the ugly plastic ileostomy bag (why wasn't someone already operating such a business?). She also bought stickers for me to dress up the bag. These helped, but I cleverly came up with my own great disguise. Throughout elementary, junior high, and high school I'd taken dance classes and still had my dance uniforms—sleek, black bodysuits. Bingo. I started wearing these bodysuits under my clothes all the time, especially whenever I was going out. It was the perfect solution. There was no possible way a "wardrobe malfunction" could reveal anything but black fabric. That alleviated a lot of stress for me.

November 19, 2002

Dear Diary,

I need to talk to more people who have been through what I have, i.e., an ostomy and surgery and Crohn's/colitis. It will be my therapy!

I didn't find anyone. I didn't know anyone else with an ostomy and I never reached out to the volunteer who'd come to visit in the hospital. Nor did it cross my mind, or was it ever suggested to me, to see a psychotherapist. I kept in touch with Julie, my friend from our days at the IWK. Our parents had made the effort to help us stay connected over the years (this was before social media). Crohn's tethered us from a distance as we led our separate lives in different school programs and in different social circles. We got together once in a while, and she had come to visit me in the hospital. But we didn't talk much about Crohn's. For me, that friendship was about finding solace in the knowledge that someone else I knew was living a life like mine, engaged in a similar battle, and going through the same things. We were simply comrades-in-Crohn's. Besides, she hadn't had the same surgery as me—yet.

I was flying on my own and doing my best to pretend nothing had happened to me at all.

CROHN'S AND COLITIS CANADA

Crohn's and Colitis Canada is the national volunteer-based charity focussed on inflammatory bowel disease and a valued resource for the community of over three hundred thousand Canadians living with IBD. It's one of the top two health charity funders of Crohn's and colitis research in the world and was founded in 1974 by parents who were driven to help their children who had a disease about which little was known.

"The whole focus was about research and awareness and—fast forward—there's been a ton of progress over forty-nine years," says Angie Specic, vice-president of marketing and communications.

According to the Crohn's and Colitis Canada website, the organization has invested over $145 million in research leading to important treatment breakthroughs and transforming the lives of people affected.

"Most of our money goes towards research, ultimately to improve lives, find cures, improve treatments, discover new things, and increase knowledge," says Specic. "We also offer programs, education, and services to support everyone affected by IBD."

Crohn's and Colitis Canada directs 78 percent of its funding toward finding a cure and improving the lives of people affected by IBD; 14 percent to administration; and 8 percent toward volunteers and services. Of the funds put toward the mission, 73 percent goes to research and 27 percent to advocacy, awareness, education, and patient programs. Revenue sources include individual giving, corporate giving, community events, the annual Gutsy Walk, and a multi-year research grant.

"Canada is home to some of the best researchers in the world," says Specic. "A lot of that is because of Crohn's and Colitis Canada supporting them, working to bring in new young talent and to support research that potentially would go unfunded."

Research initiatives currently under way include the Promoting Access and Care through Centres of Excellence (PACE) program and the Genetic, Environmental, Microbial (GEM) project (see "Research in IBD," page 80). An annual conference every November brings together the healthcare community across Canada: doctors, nurses, allied healthcare professionals, and researchers come together to share information and updates.

A report produced in 2018 (and updated in 2023) called *The Impact of Inflammatory Bowel Disease in Canada* (see page 120) offered a wide-ranging examination of the disease and its impact on Canada. It was delivered by the scientific community to Crohn's and Colitis Canada. It serves as a comprehensive, data-laden resource about the impact of Crohn's disease and ulcerative colitis across the country.

"The impact study is an important resource," says Specic. "It is a go-to for a lot of individuals…in terms of the statistics and the impact on various groups from children to seniors to patients in rural areas."

As the charity ramps up to its fiftieth anniversary in 2024, it has launched an impact strategy for 2023–2026, with objectives to accelerate the impact of research, broaden the reach of programs, drive system change, and boost awareness and understanding.

"We will build on the history and the advances that have happened over the last fifty years," says Specic. "There are far more treatments available today. There's an increase in understanding and awareness. People are talking about it more, but the work's not done."

The website (crohnsandcolitis.ca) offers resources like a learning series, webinars on diet, nutrition, and other issues, brochures and booklets covering a range of related topics, a link to Gutsy Peer Support (a service connecting individuals affected by Crohn's or colitis with each other or with support staff to get advice, emotional support, and information about living with IBD), as well as videos, articles, and reports on anything to do with IBD from research to recipes, fertility, mental health, and cannabis use.

Specic says some special webinars and content were created during Covid because of concerns about how the pandemic could impact people on medications and treatments who were immunocompromised.

"We brought together IBD experts to talk about…things like accessing infusion clinics, who's at greater risk, making sure people were on the priority list for vaccinations if they needed to be. That proved to be helpful," she says. "We helped more people during Covid than ever before. We had more web traffic; we were attracting people from around the world who were seeking content and advice during the pandemic time. We were really happy to be a valued resource for the community."

The resources are meant to help people at various stages of their IBD journey. There are summer camps for kids living with IBD (Camp Got2Go) and an IBD scholarship program to help students achieve their academic goals. MyGut is an app created by Crohn's and Colitis Canada that enables a patient to track and manage their IBD journey; GoHere is a washroom access program with an app designed to help people find available washrooms; *Talk About Guts* is Crohn's and Colitis Canada's monthly e-newsletter that keeps readers up to date on news and events and shares stories of people with IBD.

"We do a lot around social media and digital programming to make sure that our content comes up when people are seeking [a trusted source] in Canada," says Specic. "All of our content is vetted by experts. We have a scientific and medical advisory council that informs the content, so you know it's credible." There are a few key dates for Crohn's and Colitis Canada and for those impacted by IBD. November is National Crohn's and Colitis Awareness Month, a time to both raise awareness and celebrate the community. May 19 is World IBD Day, when the globe comes together in the fight against IBD. Every June the Gutsy Walk, the charity's largest fundraiser (having raised more than $50 million since its inception twenty-eight years ago), takes place across the country. "It really is a rallying point for the community to get together and connect and share and hug each other," says Specic.

Crohn's and Colitis Canada has local chapters in every province where people can connect with their community and take advantage of the opportunity to volunteer and support those living with IBD, which for many is an important way of giving back.

"It's important, the sharing of people's experiences and not everyone is willing to [share] what it means to live with this," says Specic. "Sometimes people feel a bit vulnerable, but there are so many more people now who actually are wanting to talk to media, wanting to educate [people] specifically on the severity of the disease... People don't realize that you can be in a hospital for six months, and lose a ton of weight, and have to go through these really severe surgeries just to kind of stabilize your life."

If you feel isolated you are invited to connect with your local chapter to open up the conversation. You are not alone on your IBD journey.

NAVIGATING DRUG COVERAGE

Many components of a patient's journey can be complex and stressful beyond the physical symptoms of their disease. Navigating health insurance and drug coverage is one of those components, especially when it comes to catastrophic (extremely high) drug costs.

Biologic therapies can cost thousands of dollars per treatment. However, Canadians are fortunate to have patient support programs directly through drug manufacturers for each of the biologic medications. These patient support programs provide financial assistance to help patients with their insurance co-pay and deductibles, whether administered through private or public insurance. The programs may also provide compassionate coverage of the drug if a patient's health plan will not cover the cost of the drug. The patient support programs have nurses and reimbursement specialists who can assist patients with the insurance paperwork, and who can communicate directly with the physician or nurse practitioner who prescribes the medication.

"Most patients can expect to have to pay very little, if any, out-of-pocket for their biologic medication," says Jessica Robar, nurse navigator with the NSCIBD program. Robar says she spends a fair amount of time in her role helping patients navigate their drug coverage.

Sometimes patients can be denied coverage for expensive drugs unless granted "exception status," meaning they must meet certain criteria to have the drug coverage approved. These criteria include severity of disease and other medications tried before.

"Usually the prescribers are quite familiar with the criteria required for coverage and try to keep this in mind when they prescribe the drug, unless it is something not commonly prescribed," says Robar.

"The patient support program will work with the prescriber to provide additional information and appeal letters to try and obtain coverage," says Robar. If that fails, the patient support program will likely provide the drug compassionately to the patient, especially if the patient has already started their treatment. "Most patient support programs in fact do this."

PUBLIC HEALTH INSURANCE

In Nova Scotia, any patient without private drug coverage, or with limited private drug coverage, can apply to one of several Nova Scotia Pharmacare programs. Patients are required to submit their previous year's tax information; their deductible and co-pay will be determined by their family income. For the Family Pharmacare program, the patient will only pay toward the deductible and co-pay if they need a prescription. The Seniors' Pharmacare program has an annual premium based on household income, as well as an annual co-pay. Once these amounts are maxed out and the deductible has been paid, prescriptions are fully covered, apart from the co-pay. But these deductible and co-pay amounts can be beyond the budgets of many patients.

The average cost of biologic treatment is between $21,000 and $36,000 a year for a standard dose (on Remicade, for example, a standard dose involves receiving the drug every eight weeks). If a patient requires a higher dose, the patient support program may cover the additional dosing on a compassionate basis, as Pharmacare will only cover a standard dose. Some private insurers will pay for the higher dose if a rationale is provided (for example, a patient's test results indicating they had some response to the initial treatment but the standard dose is not enough to be fully effective).

In some cases, a drug is not listed on the Pharmacare formulary for the treatment of IBD. The formulary details which drugs and devices are eligible under the Pharmacare programs.

"Patients on Pharmacare may get the drug compassionately from the manufacturer," says Robar. "I know that our public insurance program will take into account reports from the Canadian Agency for Drugs and Technologies in Health. This agency will review drugs in detail and take many factors into consideration when making recommendations."

BIOSIMILARS

Robar says many patients are now switching to a biosimilar form of their biologic due to changes to the biologic medications that insurance companies—both public and private—will cover. Biosimilars are drugs that have been proven to be highly similar (but not exactly the same) to the original biologic medications; they are emerging on the market as biologic patents expire, but not every patient is comfortable making this switch.

"For a non-medical switch to be approved by Health Canada, studies must show that there are no clinical differences or changes in outcome between a patient taking a biosimilar drug and one taking the original biologic," explains Robar. She says switching to biosimilars will save insurance companies and public health insurance plans like Pharmacare millions of dollars because biosimilars, like generic drugs, cost less to make. The average cost for biosimilar treatment is about $13,000 to 16,000 per year, which is nearly half the cost of the originator drugs.

Robar says this substantial cost savings will give insurance plans (public and private) the ability to afford coverage for other, very expensive, medications, including new biologics that will come to market that don't yet have cost-saving biosimilar options. Theoretically, could actually improve and expand the treatment options they will cover for IBD. It remains to be seen. This switch has happened with public insurance programs in most Canadian provinces. The government of Nova Scotia expanded the use of biosimilar medications in Nova Scotia Pharmacare programs. As of February 2023, Humira and Remicade are not covered by Pharmacare unless an exemption is granted, because a biosimilar version is approved and available. A prescriber can apply for an exemption for clinical reasons. If this exemption is not approved, or if the patient doesn't qualify for an exemption, coverage of the original biologic medication will end, essentially forcing the patient to switch to the cheaper medication.

There are certain instances where an exception to a a forced switch to a biosimilar may be considered. Exceptions could include if a patient is in a current flare of symptoms that is not under control, is pregnant, or if multiple biologics have failed and the current drug is their last available option.

"I believe that if an appeal failed or was denied, the patient would be left with the option to cover the cost of the drug themselves or to choose an alternate drug that might be covered, meaning switching to a totally different medication, which could be a considerable risk, or stopping the drug if they do not want to switch," says Robar.

In my case, my small, private health insurance plan will not cover the cost of my biologic drug treatment. My income bracket leaves the co-pay and deductibles through Nova Scotia Pharmacare too high to afford—plus I'm not comfortable switching to a biosimilar option due to the severity of my disease. Because of this, the manufacturer of my drug has granted me compassionate coverage and provided me with a compassionate supply of the drug, leaving me with no out-of-pocket expense for this medication. This decision is re-evaluated every year.

OTHER RESOURCES

There are some occasions when a patient simply cannot afford a drug. "We usually only see this when a patient is not on a biologic," says Robar. Examples of these expensive drugs are some types of steroids, some 5-ASAs, and some antibiotics. The expense ranges from $200 to $400 for a month's supply.

If a medication is not covered, says Robar, "we can do a few things. We can consider prescribing a different medication, see if samples can be obtained from the manufacturer, see if the manufacturer has compassionate programs or assistance cards, or see if there is a pharmacy that might have different pricing than the patient's usual pharmacy."

Another resource Robar suggests that people might not know about is calling 211, which is Canada's primary source of information for government and community-based, non-clinical health and social services. "They will point you in the direction of any community resources that might be able to help you," she says.

Robar also emphasizes that patients should not be afraid to tell their physician or nurse practitioner they cannot afford a medication. "Pharmacists may also be able to help if they are knowledgeable about resources and can send communication back to the physicians regarding alternate options."

DIET, NUTRITION, AND IBD

Crohn's disease and ulcerative colitis affect the body's ability to digest food and absorb nutrients properly. Crohn's can affect anywhere along the gastrointestinal tract, also known as the digestive system, with inflammation occurring anywhere from "your gums to your bum," as the IBD catch-phrase goes, preventing absorption of nutrients from foods you eat. Ulcerative colitis typically causes inflammation only in the colon, where water is absorbed from food. That inflammation prevents that absorption, meaning stools can become watery.

While diet alone does not cause IBD, it certainly plays a role in a patient's experience with IBD. Their diet will likely vary at times, changing when the disease flares up and again when it is in remission.

Mallory O'Neill is a registered dietitian who has spent time working with IBD patients in the gastroenterology clinic in Halifax. The main referrals she receives are for patients dealing with unintentional weight loss, food avoidance, over-restricting (meaning not eating enough), and malnutrition. Often, patients come to her while they are experiencing a flare-up of their disease, and she continues to monitor them when they are in remission.

"I'll chat with patients if they want to discuss their diet and ways to potentially help prevent flares," says O'Neill. She helps patients design a healthy, varied diet to prevent further weight loss or to put on weight and to manage symptoms. If patients are experiencing a lot of diarrhea, gas, bloating, and abdominal pain, she helps find ways to meet their nutritional needs while managing those symptoms. O'Neill also sees patients with ostomies and with feeding tubes to help them manage ways to live and eat well.

There is no one-size-fits-all diet for IBD. "It's very individual, and that's where it's nice to have one-on-one time to get to know the patient and what they are eating," says O'Neill. "Everyone is different. People often have foods they find they don't tolerate or foods they avoid. One person may not tolerate something and another person tolerates it well."

She does not advise patients to follow a specific diet, but if they are in a flare with active inflammation and they are experiencing symptoms like diarrhea, frequent bowel movements, urgency, abdominal pain, bloating, and gas she will have them focus on a low–insoluble fibre diet. "Limiting things like nuts and seeds, peelings on fruits and vegetables, whole grains, any raw vegetables, things like that," says O'Neill. "But if diarrhea is a problem, we'll chat about adding in more foods that can help bulk up stool—so, depending on the patient and their symptoms, usually two sources of bulk-forming foods with each meal, one to two with snacks. Things like applesauce, bananas, white potatoes or sweet potatoes (peeled and cooked), white pastas, white bread, smooth peanut butter."

Another important point that O'Neill raises with her patients is their increased need for protein to help repair tissue, especially when in a flare. She says it can be difficult for patients to focus on protein. "A common thing I see with a lot of people is difficulty tolerating red meats," she says. "We'll chat about ways to incorporate more protein and make sure they're eating enough protein to meet their needs. Sometimes it may [require] adding supplements; it could be a protein powder, it could be an oral nutrition supplement. Fluids can be easier at times, so…protein drinks can be a way to do that."

When a patient is in remission and they want to eat an overall healthy diet, O'Neill will talk to them about the Mediterranean diet, "which is basically a healthy balanced diet with plant-based proteins, fruits and vegetables, whole grains, things like that," she says. "If someone is in remission and not having a lot of symptoms, we'll chat about having a higher-fibre diet because that is recommended to help to prevent future flare-ups, unless of course they have strictures, then we wouldn't. We would do a long-term low-fibre diet."

A stricture is a narrowing in the intestine, usually as a result of a buildup of scar tissue caused by repeated cycles of inflammation and healing in the lining of the intestine.

When a patient who has no stricturing is not in an active flare-up, O'Neill will talk with them about finding a good balance of healthy fats and increasing variety in their diet, especially if they were over-restricting certain foods while they were sick. She explains that, when not in a flare, patients can often eat those foods again. "They aren't going to have the same tolerance issues," she says. If they are trying to gain weight back, she'll incorporate high-calorie, high-protein foods. It's common to experiment with elements of various diets to find out what helps.

"In terms of specific diets, like the Crohn's Disease Exclusion Diet [CDED], it's often something the patient requests," says O'Neill. "They've heard about it and want to try it, or a doctor might recommend it if medications aren't working for them. It's not often that I necessarily recommend it to a lot of patients, because it's super, super restrictive, but I have seen it be helpful for some people to maintain remission and in some cases induce remission, so it is an option. Because a lot of the patients I see are already over-restricting, have lost weight, have a really poor appetite, it's sort of contraindicated in some of those cases."

According to information on the Crohn's and Colitis Canada website, the CDED is "based on excluding elements of the Western diet that are associated with causing inflammation and changing the environment of the gut. It combines whole foods with partial enteral nutrition [see sidebar] in two stages, the first more restrictive than the second in order to induce remission." The website also shares how a randomized controlled trial has shown that the CDED with partial enteral nutrition "is effective to induce remission in children with mild-to-moderate Crohn's disease and helps maintain remission up to twelve weeks. Studies in adults with Crohn's disease show promising results, and clinical trials are ongoing."

O'Neill says the diet also has a long-term maintenance phase that is somewhat more liberalized, with "cheat days" while still being fairly restrictive, with an additional supplement suggested that is very expensive. Oral nutrition supplements can be used instead.

"There is also exclusive enteral nutrition, which I have had a couple patients do, but really the research is in pediatrics, and I see adults," says O'Neill. "It's really difficult to not eat for that extended period of time and only take a formula, so

Exclusive enteral nutrition (EEN), also known as tube feeding, is explained on the Crohn's and Colitis Canada website as "a type of treatment that includes a nutritional formula taken by mouth or by placing a tube in the nose or in the gut. EEN delivers daily nutrients to the body in liquid form and helps get your disease under control. It also helps with catch-up weight gain, optimizing growth potential, healing the lining of the intestines, reducing swelling, and improving symptoms, with very [few] side effects."

it's hard for adults to do, but it can certainly help to induce remission and bring down inflammation if someone's able to adhere to it. That's the challenge. It's about what's feasible and realistic for the patient."

Another specific diet, the low-FODMAP diet, isn't studied much in the context of IBD but is in relation to IBS (Irritable Bowel Syndrome). O'Neill does have patients with IBD and likely underlying IBS, so the diet can be helpful for them in managing the IBS symptoms, but it isn't known to help battle inflammation. The diet is challenging to follow because many foods contain FODMAPs.

O'Neill says limiting processed foods is important when you're in remission, but that can be difficult to do when you're sick. "When you're in a flare there's just so much going on, so much contributing to [whether you are] able to eat enough, [that] I wouldn't focus on that a whole lot. We're just trying to make sure you're eating enough and getting protein." But when you're in remission, she says, limiting food additives and having a healthy, varied diet with fruits and vegetables and higher fibre can be helpful, although it may not prevent flare-ups.

When it comes to diet and IBD, O'Neill says it's important to be wary of unsolicited advice and to take careful note of where information comes from.

"What works for someone else may not work for you. If

> FODMAP stands for fermentable oligosaccharides, disaccharides, monosaccharides, and polyols, which are short-chain carbohydrates (sugars) that the small intestine absorbs poorly. Some of the foods to avoid on the FODMAP diet are broccoli, Brussels sprouts, cabbage, eggplant, garlic, onions, and breads and crackers made from gluten sources like wheat or rye.

anyone says there's a cure by eating a certain way, be careful. [And] be very wary of what you see online.... A lot of it isn't necessarily evidence-based. Seeking professional help is important."

O'Neill recommends seeing a dietitian who can work with you individually. She also points to the Gastrointestinal Society for helpful videos from dietitians and notes that Crohn's and Colitis Canada also has a lot of informative resources, including webinars.

"It can be overwhelming, so if you're in a flare [and] thinking it's because of things you were eating, know that's not the case," she says. "Do the best you can...and stop being hard on yourself, because it can be a challenge navigating everything."

MY STORY:
FROM REVERSAL TO
RESEARCH STUDY
(2002–2007)

December 24, 2002

Dear Diary,

I am happy and healthy, and that's what counts! It's Christmas Eve! I'm so excited! The feeling doesn't change, every year the night before Christmas, I feel the same way. I can't wait!!

It was three months post-surgery and things were going well. Really well. I was getting on with my life. I hadn't missed a beat that first semester, proudly scoring higher than Matt in our mid-term exams—despite having missed most of the classes that term—using his notes to study. My academic adviser had encouraged me to drop out of my courses and catch up later, but there was no way I was being left a semester behind my friends. Recovery was physically simple as I slowly gained my strength back. Mentally, I'd already packed my bags for the next surgery. Most importantly, I was finally feeling well. Despite the bag on my side, I was granted a new-found freedom from illness. The stoma didn't represent illness to me; it represented recovery.

I turned twenty. Matt and I properly celebrated our one-year anniversary. The surgery hadn't scared him off. He wasn't going anywhere; he was just happy I was healthy. My priorities shifted to more pressing matters, like what to wear to the Halloween party at our campus pub. Life became about juggling a part-time job, university classes, and a social life, along with taking care of my new accessory.

February 3, 2003

Dear Diary,

I really want to have the reversal surgery. I'm really scared about it. What if I make the wrong choice? I suppose the doctors know what's best. I've been doing 150 crunches every night. I really want a nice stomach to show off when I get rid of the pouch. I'm back at dance class now, and have been walking. I need to get my energy back up. I still get so out of breath coming up the stairs. I'm excited. About life in general.

I did waver slightly in making the decision about my next move. I was so healthy and feeling good, living my life. Did I want to rock the boat and wind up right back where I started? I knew what I *wanted* to do; I was just frightened that having the colectomy reversed would be the wrong choice. But I knew deep down I had to at least give it a try and I wanted to be fit and healthy when I did it.

In preparation, I had a follow-up appointment with my surgeon. He agreed it was worth trying and that it would be fine to go ahead. I had no signs of disease or inflammation anywhere else. There were a few surgical options but the best was an ileorectal anastomosis. They'd reconnect my small bowel to what was left of my large bowel. They'd take the five centimetres of colon I had left at the very bottom (keep in mind a colon is five feet long) and reattach it to my ileum, the stoma sticking out of my side. Everything would be back on the inside—hooked up again.

"In the long term, you may require removal of the rectum and a permanent ileostomy, but this will depend on how active your Crohn's is in the future," my surgeon told me. "The surgery could last you up to twenty years"—far enough into the future that I decided I could deal with that tidbit of information later. He warned I could flare up all over again, but knew I could without this surgery, too. I'd made the decision back in September and I hadn't changed my mind. If the surgery was an option, it was the option I was going for. If I didn't need the ileostomy, the ileostomy was going.

Booking the reconnection surgery was a very simple process. I was given a phone number to call; the clerk gave me the first few available dates, which were in about two months. I picked April 24, after my exams were finished. I would use the summer to recover. It was as simple as that. I was given an appointment time and prep instructions.

March 2, 2003

Dear Diary,

I booked my surgery—the 24th of April. The surgeon thinks it's worth a shot! Oh, I hope it works!! Please! It's going to hurt and I hate staying in the hospital...but I'm willing to try. I haven't yet accepted having this ileostomy forever. No. I want it to work so badly!!

It was an incredibly different experience to walk into the hospital for a *planned* major surgery, as opposed to winding up in the OR after spending time as an in-patient. The first time, I had been wheeled away to the OR on a stretcher. This time, I arrived at the hospital with my mother in the wee hours of the morning; I checked in, changed into a johnny shirt (all my belongings went into a plastic bag I towed along with me) and sat in the waiting room until they called my name. I walked into the OR, hopped on the table, and lay back, waiting to be put to sleep—knowing what to expect.

"Next you can get some plastic surgery, take care of that scar, and you'll be back in your bikini on the beach," a nurse said to me as I lay there, waiting for the surgery to begin.

The nurse meant well. I just nodded along in agreement. But it struck me. A girl can't wear a bikini with a scar? Sure, I'd been working on my stomach by doing crunches, but I'd have to have more surgery just to put on a bikini? That didn't seem right.

It wasn't the only slight I heard that day. "You were so nice and tiny for the first surgery," Dr. Jamieson told me at my bedside after the surgery. "This time I had to cut in much higher." He wasn't being insensitive, just matter-of-fact—as if he had to justify his work, and it was my fault it wasn't to his standard. I wondered if I was supposed to apologize.

I had gone into the first surgery weighing 90 pounds. I was *literally* wasting away. And yes, I had a neat little scar that started curving just around the top of my belly button, running down to my pubic bone. For this surgery I went in at a healthy 120 pounds. This time, the incision started about eight inches above my belly button and down to the pubic bone. Near it was a smaller incision about two inches long and half an inch wide, the shadow of my ostomy.

In one way that OR nurse had been right. I was back in my bikini on the beach in no time. But I was rocking my scars. I loved my scars. Unlike the stigma-fuelled ileostomy bag, I loved showing them off. I loved answering questions about them. My scars told a great story. With the surgeries behind me, I was so proud to have won that fight. The scars were my battle wounds.

May 30, 2003

Dear Diary,

I'm really, really happy I had the surgery. It went quite well; the recovery was long, though, like a month. I guess I am still recovering. A few minor problems, but so far so good! It's weird though! Sometimes I think it's strange now without it, sometimes I find it hard to believe I had it!! I don't really like thinking about it a lot. I was in hospital only for a week, and the "roommates" were all right. I spent a lot of time at home watching TV. My scar is a pain, still draining and stuff. I hope, really hope, I stay well. I don't ever want to go through that again! Please, not again. I'm going to watch what I eat though. Big time. I want to look, feel, and be healthy.

The second time around, recovering from surgery was harder. Perhaps it was because I'd gone into it feeling well, so having to recover brought me down a bit. The first time, I'd been so sick going into surgery that I felt immediately better when I came out of it. This time, my incision didn't heal properly, and I had to deal with an infection, but I was soon on the mend.

In June, I got the all-clear at a follow-up appointment. I was feeling well, having no Crohn's symptoms, and hadn't required any medications since the first surgery in September. I was generally well and stable. The old ileostomy site and scars were looking healthy. Like a gold star at the bottom of my report: *In summary, Ms. McLeod is a 20-year-old female with Crohn's colitis who is currently in remission after ileorectal anastomosis in April of this year.*

A fabulous summer passed by. I was working part-time and having fun taking carefree adventures around Nova Scotia filled with tidal-bore rafting, swimming, hiking, and camping. I was making up for all the time I'd spent the previous summer doing things while I was sick and in pain. Matt and I took our first trip together. We lived it up in Toronto—shopping, taking in a Blue Jays game, trying every ride at Canada's Wonderland, going to a Bryan Adams concert, the Canadian National Exhibition (CNE), and taking in *The Lion King* musical.

When we started back at university that fall, I was healthy and happy. Finally, I could focus my attention on the typical pressures most young adults were faced with at that time in their lives: studying, working, navigating new social circles, building a resumé, and making plans for the future.

February 23, 2004
Patient Name: McLeod, Heather
Report sent to: Dr. David T. MacNeil, family physician

I had the pleasure of seeing Heather today in the GI clinic on the 23rd of February. As you are aware, she has had a total colectomy with an ileoanal anastomosis. This was nearly a year ago.

Heather has been perfectly well with no medications.

I do not think there is any reason to change anything with Heather at this point and I will see her in one year's time in follow-up.

I do not think any other intervention is necessary.

Yours sincerely,
Munaa Khaliq-Kareemi, MD, FRCPC
Attending Staff, Dept. of Med (Gastroenterology)

An order for follow-up in one year felt like winning a golden ticket. I was on my way, symptom-free and in complete remission. Despite the opinion of my surgeon that I could flare again—I was never misled—naïveté kicked in. I kind of just figured *my* Crohn's wouldn't be so chronic. I'd had my turn, I'd done it all, I'd paid my dues, and I was off that path—my golden ticket guiding me on to the next pain-free chapter of my life.

Nine months later, as I was preparing to leave for England, I started to run into trouble. On November 12, 2004, I would be heading off for an exciting internship in the UK as part of my journalism degree. I'd be working at a women's magazine called *Company*, a glossy publication much like *Cosmopolitan*. A once-in-a-lifetime, can't-believe-this-is-happening kind of opportunity. I had no room for unforeseen circumstances. But on November 4, I found myself back at the GI clinic.

The disease was starting to stir, waking from far too short a slumber. Slowly but surely symptoms started creeping back into my life. I started feeling pain in my belly after I ate. I was back on alert. Given that I didn't have much of a colon left, the official diagnosis was confirmed. It couldn't be ulcerative colitis, which is inflammation of the colon. It was full-blown Crohn's, which can attack the entire digestive system from the "gums to the bum." Six years after my initial diagnosis, the pathology conducted after the surgery confirmed it. What had been thought to be ulcerative colitis ended up being a special blend of Crohn's and colitis.

A flexible sigmoidoscopy is a procedure in which a sigmoidoscope or scope—a narrow, flexible fibre optic tube about 60 cm long with a light and a tiny camera on one end—is used to look inside the rectum and lower colon.

Dr. Kareemi felt a flexible sigmoidoscopy was necessary in short order to see what was going on. He rushed me in for the procedure, which confirmed inflammation at the anastomosis (the spot where my small bowel had been reconnected to my large bowel) and a fistula—an abnormal, infected, tunnel-like passageway leading off from what was remaining of my colon—that was causing pain.

I was prescribed a cocktail of antibiotics, ciprofloxacin (Cipro) and metronidazole (Flagyl), just before heading off to London. It crossed my mind that maybe I shouldn't go. What if my health spiralled? But I brushed the thought aside. Something bad could happen to *anyone*. I was determined to go. The Flagyl left a gross metallic taste in my mouth, but it helped.

I lucked out. I got through the six-week internship happy and healthy. It was my first taste of living away from home—on my own and on another continent at that—and I enjoyed every second of it. Eternally grateful everything had gone smoothly, I returned home and eventually finished the course of medication—and then the symptoms promptly returned.

On February 18, 2005, I was back at the all-too-familiar GI clinic once again—just a few days ahead of the date that had been scheduled for my one-year follow-up. I hadn't quite made it.

Dr. Kareemi put me back on Cipro and added another medication called budesonide (Entocort) to try and settle the inflammation. Entocort is a type of corticosteroid used to help reduce inflammation in different parts of the body—better than having to take prednisone, but not without its own set of unwanted side effects. He suggested that we may need to start thinking about immunosuppressive therapy to control the Crohn's. Because azathioprine (Imuran), the next drug in line, caused me to have elevated liver enzymes in the past and I couldn't tolerate the drug, we'd have to bypass that one and consider something called methotrexate—a drug often used to fight cancer but also sometimes used to treat Crohn's.

For the next six weeks I took the Entocort for the inflammation, plus another round of antibiotics, healing the fistula completely. The report from an appointment in April said: *Has been doing very well since last appt in February with Dr. Kareemi.* Despite the recent scope showing active inflammation, a fistula, and two new prescription medications, I was apparently doing "very well."

After stopping the antibiotic, I continued on the Entocort. At any recurrence of the fistula (with symptoms of pain, fever, chills), I had to restart the Cipro and think about starting immunosuppressive therapy. Sure enough, come June, the fistula recurred. Dr. Kareemi suggested it was time to go on methotrexate.

I now had active disease around the anastomosis and a recurrent fistula. I was slowly being called to stand on guard, struggling against this unpredictable disease. I'd managed to keep illness at bay with an antibiotic here and there topped up by another medication, almost-but-not-quite heading back into full battle mode. Now I was being thrust into the world of new and nagging symptoms, making my way through a whole new set of meds again.

I was freshly graduated from university and had to navigate a new professional life at my first full-time job while managing my shaky health. I had my first apartment in the city, living with my best friend Christina. She was well aware of my health status so there were no secrets there. Our apartment was conveniently located right between the hospital and the university office where I was working—a short walk to work and to doctors' appointments.

Dr. Kareemi made all the arrangements for me to start methotrexate but sadly wouldn't be able to see me through it. He was leaving town, moving out west to take a job in Calgary. He booked me an appointment to follow up in four weeks with a nurse practitioner at the GI clinic.

I needed to learn how to inject myself with the new medication. Near the end of June, my mom and I set off for the Patient and Family Learning Centre at the VG. I hadn't flown entirely away from the nest and my mother had come to learn how to do it as well, in case I ever needed her to step in and help me. The nurse educator shared information on the medication and its side effects. Methotrexate is a chemotherapy agent and immune-system suppressant. It is used to treat cancer (in much higher doses), inflammatory conditions like Crohn's, other autoimmune diseases, and ectopic pregnancies. It slows down your body's immune system and helps reduce inflammation. The long list of possible side effects include nausea, vomiting, stomach pain, diarrhea, hair loss, tiredness, dizziness, chills, and headaches—ironically, a lot of the same symptoms caused by Crohn's disease. And because the medication suppresses the immune system, it leaves users at risk of infection.

We learned about proper storage of the medication and supplies, preparation and administration of the medication, and its safe disposal. I'd need to inject it into my abdomen once a week. The medication came in a tiny glass vial. We learned how to draw the medication up with a syringe, tap on the side to remove any tiny air bubbles, then switch the cap to a needle. I had to wipe a spot on my abdomen with an alcohol swab, pinch the flesh on my stomach, jab myself with the needle, and slowly inject the medication. Once finished, everything would go into a big yellow biohazard container that I'd return to the pharmacy once it was full. We practiced with saline, injecting it into mounds of silicone. Model students, my mom and I learned everything we needed to know with ease and were sent on our way.

I handled the injections myself with no problem, collecting little poke-marks on my abdomen that would itch and sting. But seven months later I'd had enough of the lingering flu-like symptoms the medication caused, and they seemed to be increasing. A month after the calendar ticked over to 2006, I stopped taking the medication altogether. I now had a new GI specialist, Dr. Dana Farina, a young, friendly, compassionate, and approachable doctor, with whom I had a great rapport. I stopped the methotrexate, and after a month he suggested trying again, this time on a lower dose. I agreed, and we came up with a plan to slowly increase the dose as far as I could tolerate it. My symptoms waxed and waned, sometimes stable, sometimes flaring, always teetering just a little to either side of decent baseline levels. I didn't know if these symptoms were side effects from the drug or if it was my Crohn's.

I stayed well enough to enjoy a whirlwind two-week holiday with Matt to the UK, where we met many of his friends and relatives in England and Scotland. We snuck a beach holiday into the mix, jetting off to Portugal on a cheap flight for a few days of relaxation. My health was not at its best, but nowhere near its worst.

A few months later, on September 19, 2006, Matt popped the question at a beautifully scenic look-off on the Cabot Trail. It was a total surprise. We'd booked a quiet weekend away because we knew it was going to be busy around the city with various concerts and sporting events going on, plus all the university students flooding back into town. While the proposal itself was a surprise, it wasn't surprising. Everyone had seen this next step coming. We were simply meant to be. Some may have thought we were too young to be engaged at twenty-three. But we were best friends, in love. Why would we part ways to see what else was out there when we were so happy together? We'd already been through huge ordeals with my surgeries and handled them well, so we'd checked the "in sickness and in health" vow off the list already. We couldn't wait to get married. We had the guest list completed before we even made it back to the city, planning for a summer wedding the following year.

Later that fall, I decided to drop the methotrexate altogether once again. The nausea and the constant feeling of general malaise had become too much. But the following January, February, and March were rough.

Right after the holidays, in early 2007, I gave notice that I was going to leave the university office where I was working; I was taking a position as associate editor at a local lifestyle magazine where I'd been freelancing on the side. The magazine was changing hands and the editing position was my dream job. But two days after I gave my notice, I felt horribly sick. My symptoms had crept up on me slowly, but now they were to the point where I was unable to work at all. Though I'd just given my notice, I had to take sick leave to get through my remaining time in that position.

Unfortunately, at the last minute, the magazine deal fell through, and I had to rescind my resignation at my office job even though I was still off on sick leave—which surely seemed suspicious. I was also trying to stay on top of my wedding plans, which is stressful at the best of times. I was so unwell I had to go stay at my parents' house. At my doctor's suggestion we tried the low dose of methotrexate one more time.

A few weeks later, still just as sick, the same job opportunity came up with the magazine. A new deal was being worked out, and once again I had the opportunity to apply for my dream job. But the new owner was in Toronto, and they wanted to meet me. I had to decline the first invitation to travel to Toronto because there was no way I could manage it. I told them I was sick at the time, but they didn't know to what extent. They asked me to go a week or so later. I knew I had to do it or risk losing an amazing opportunity. After having spent weeks sick in bed, I mustered up the energy and flew to Toronto for meetings. I was wined and dined, and no one knew I was in a horrible flare and felt like garbage. But there was no way I was letting Crohn's stand in my way of securing that job. Thankfully, everything worked out and I signed a contract with the magazine. The best part—I would work from home, which would be ideal in terms of helping me get a handle on my health.

By then I'd developed an aversion to the whole process with methotrexate. Just the idea of injecting myself with a needle made me feel nauseous. I also started thinking a lot about the long-term effects, and I didn't like the prospect of those either, especially the possibility of liver damage. I just did not enjoy being on that medication. My quality of life was being affected and I knew it was not how I wanted to continue. I'd been yo-yoing on and off the methotrexate. Without it, my Crohn's flares and symptoms got worse. On it, I felt lousy *and* the flare symptoms, while slightly improved, still lingered.

Knowing how much I was not enjoying my treatment plan, Dr. Farina suggested I consider joining a trial study the hospital was running for a new drug called adalimumab (Humira). Humira is a biologic drug (meaning it's produced with live cells) that acts as an immunosuppressant to help stop inflammation in the body. Tumour necrosis factor–alpha (TNF–α) is a cytokine protein in your body that causes inflammation. In a healthy person, TNF helps the body fight off infections. Inflammation can be a good thing; it happens when your immune system is fighting a possible threat. An overactive immune system may attack healthy parts of the body, leading to too much TNF. In people with inflammatory bowel diseases like Crohn's and colitis and other autoimmune disorders, high levels of TNF in the blood can cause unnecessary inflammation.

Anti-TNF antibodies, or TNF inhibitors, such as adalimumab (Humira) and infliximab (Remicade, another biologic medication) target and block the action of TNF–α in your body, helping stop inflammation; this can make the disease go away and allow your body to heal. Anti-TNF antibodies can be very effective at settling down the disease. However, they aren't for everybody—they are powerful, and come with risk of infection or rare tumour growth.

The research study suggested for me was being offered by the hospital to find better ways of caring for people with Crohn's disease. The goal of the trial was to find out if adalimumab was useful for people with Crohn's disease. The open-label clinical trial was set to start over the next couple of weeks, and it was my doctor's hope to get me enrolled for a chance to try a different treatment. He gave me literature about the study and left me to think about it.

Why Is This Trial Being Done?

The study is with a drug called adalimumab. It is being studied in the treatment for Crohn's disease. Crohn's disease is a chronic inflammatory disease involving the digestive tract. There is no cure for Crohn's disease. Current treatment is aimed at managing the symptoms of inflammation that occur with this disease. The body's immune system (natural defence) is believed to be involved in causing Crohn's disease. Immunosuppressive drugs (drugs that change the immune system), such as Imuran, 6MP, and methotrexate, are used to treat Crohn's disease in patients that do not respond to aminosalicylates (like Salofalk) and short-term corticosteroid therapy (like prednisone). Some patients need several medications to control their symptoms.

Current available medications often have unwanted side effects or are not completely effective in all patients. There is a need for new treatments for Crohn's disease and therapies with few side effects that are able to increase the amount of time that patients are free of symptoms or have only mild symptoms. Adalimumab may help patients with Crohn's disease that have not had complete relief of their symptoms with current available medications.

I absolutely fit the bill. This type of treatment was being developed for people like me. I'd cycled through all the meds; the immunosuppressive drugs—azathioprine and methotrexate—the aminosalicylates like Salofalk, Pentasa, and Asacol, and too many short and long-term corticosteroid therapies. They all either came with unwanted side effects or were not completely effective. Nothing could control my symptoms for any length of time.

February 28, 2007
Patient Name: Fegan, Heather
Report sent to: Dr. David T. MacNeil, family physician

We all met with Heather today to review options. Basically, at this point, she has three choices. The first one being a surgery and an ileostomy. Heather is not interested in surgery at this point. Her second two choices are both medical therapy. They include treatment with Remicade in combination with methotrexate or treatment with Humira, humanized anti-TNF antibody, through a clinical trial. Heather has read and researched both of these medications and she seems much more interested in the Humira today.

Both the potential benefits as well as the potential risks were reviewed with Heather today and I think she is going to go ahead with the study.

We will book her back in the IBD clinic in a week's time for initial study screening.

Yours sincerely,
Dana M. Farina, MD, FRCPC
Attending Staff, Dept. of Med (Gastroenterology)

This type of newer immunosuppressive therapy was the type of treatment I'd had my surgery to avoid in the first place— experimental drugs still being studied, long-term side effects unknown. But it had been nearly two years since my surgery and Humira was showing positive results in patients with IBD. I didn't really have anything else to try, so without trying to overthink things, I joined the study.

I had to have blood tests, a chest X-ray, and a tuberculosis test, all looking for any evidence of current infection. It was important to rule out any kind of infection that could run rampant when my immune system was suppressed by the drug. I passed all the tests and met all the criteria.

It was official: I was enrolled in the study.

RESEARCH IN IBD

Researchers all over the world are focussed on improving the lives of people affected by IBD and are searching for causes, and ultimately a cure, for Crohn's disease and ulcerative colitis.

Crohn's and Colitis Canada, the national charity focussed on IBD, has invested over $145 million in research which has led to important breakthroughs in genetics, gut microbes, and in our understanding of inflammation and cell repair. That research has laid the groundwork for new and better treatments and for improved symptom management strategies.

One of the research initiatives currently underway is the Promoting Access and Care through Centres of Excellence (PACE) program, which brings together leading IBD centres from across the country to improve health outcomes, address gaps in care, and drive change and improvement in the system around caring for IBD.

Another is the Genetic, Environmental, Microbial (GEM) Project, a global research study seeking to uncover possible triggers of Crohn's disease. Initiated in 2008, the GEM Project recruited first-degree relatives of Crohn's patients to be monitored to see if they would develop the disease. Researchers tracked their diet, immune function, intestinal barrier, microbiome, genetics, and environment. So far, researchers have discovered certain changes in blood and tissue that appear more frequently in the participants who developed Crohn's disease.

Dr. Jennifer Jones of the NSCIBD program at the QEII says Nova Scotia is quite active in industry-funded clinical trials. "New medications...that are very promising are in the latter stages of study, with lots of trials ongoing and more coming up. There's lots of hope there."

WHAT TO EXPECT FROM A CLINICAL TRIAL

A clinical trial is a study in which people with a specific illness volunteer to test out a new drug. Clinical trials take place in four phases:

- Phase 1: Administration of an experimental drug to a small group of people for the first time to assess the drug's safety, ideal dosage, and side effects;
- Phase 2: The drug is given to a larger group of people (a hundred or more) to assess similar concerns, as well as the drug's efficacy;
- Phase 3: A larger group (a thousand or more) receive the drug and assess it for efficacy, side effects, and how it compares to commonly used treatments;
- Phase 4: After the drug is approved and is on the market, trials take place to gather information on the long-term benefits and risks.

(Source: Health Canada)

Shari Smith is the research manager in gastroenterology research at the Centre for Clinical Research at the QEII Health Sciences Centre. She heads up the clinical trials for various pharmaceuticals aimed at treating Crohn's disease and ulcerative colitis. She says a practitioner may feel their patient would benefit from one of the studies and offer that as an option for the patient. At that point, the Centre for Clinical Research would take over and send the patient the informed consent form, which would list all the risks and benefits, as well as information about what the trial is for and how many people are in the trial. "Then we'd sit down and have that informed discussion in case they had any questions [about] the risks that may be associated with it, if any," says Smith.

Most of the drugs being tested through the Centre for Clinical Research are in Phase 3 trials. By the time a drug hits Phase 3 it's already gone through most of the regulatory bodies and the research ethics board has already approved it. "They will assign whether it's a mild-risk, moderate-risk, or high-risk study. We don't normally do high-risk studies where I am," she says.

The centre's earliest clinical trials were typically presented to patients who had very few other options, but that has changed. "Now [trials are] presented in everyday care—whether [patients] are newly diagnosed or twenty-five years with the disease," says Smith. In the interest of safety, there are strict inclusion and exclusion criteria for trials. "If your hemoglobin was way too low or your lymphocytes are [low] we're not going to subject you to a clinical trial until you're stable."

Smith says the Centre for Clinical Research usually has a few studies going on at a time for both Crohn's and ulcerative colitis. When a study starts, researchers could be looking for three hundred to fifteen hundred patients worldwide. "We always try at least to get five patients locally, hopefully more. For some studies we've had up to thirty patients." The trial drug is provided at no cost, and expenses like parking and travel are covered.

When the trial ends, patients who've had positive results may have the option of continuing with the medication once it's on the market. "Normally after you've been through a trial, you're not going to turn around and pay out-of-pocket for it. There are usually programs to cover it," says Smith.

But in other cases, patients may be disappointed to learn they can't continue with a treatment. "Sometimes a trial will end and, unfortunately, [the drug is] just not going to go to market," she says. "The patient would be sent back to their specialist, who they see all through the trial, and would be put on something comparable, if possible."

The goal of this research is to try to find new treatments that are safe and effective. "It's not a one-size-fits-all," says Smith.

"What works really well for one person may not work really well for another person. If you find something that really works well for you, that's great. It's trying to gather more options for patients with Crohn's."

INVESTIGATOR-INITIATED RESEARCH

Dr. Jones says there is also a lot of activity on the investigator-initiated side of research. A lot of the focus is on studying and evaluating models of care, innovations in care, and how to best implement and sustain these in Nova Scotia and other provinces.

Mental health interventions like IBD Strong—the program to address the needs of someone living with IBD in relation to mental health—is one example.

Implementing an externally facing nurse navigational role to overcome access inequity for marginalized populations, in collaboration with PACE program, is another. "We're starting in the Northern zone in Nova Scotia and then rolling that out gradually," says Jones.

Another strategy that Jones is working on with her colleague, Dr. Michael Stewart, is called Gut Link, an initiative to implement ways to give primary care practitioners more "ready-access" support while their patients await specialty care.

Jones is also working on a vaccination program. "Primary care is not always confident with their knowledge base in relation to managing vaccines and individuals on immunosuppressants, for example," she says. "Gastroenterologists may or may not have much vaccine knowledge and may or may not feel that it's their role to screen for vaccine-preventable illness and then advise on and implement vaccines. So it kind of leaves the person living with IBD in a care gap."

Jones is engaging care providers, nurses, doctors, and patients to try to understand what their needs are in order to best design a program that ensures that consensus guidelines for vaccine-preventable illness are consistently implemented in practice.

All of these are just a few of the research initiatives seeking a cure and exploring ways to improve the lives of people affected by IBD. Jones says there's much more she would like to do.

MY STORY:
TRYING HUMIRA
(2007–2008)

In March 2007, I took my first loading dose to get started on Humira. The loading dose is a higher initial dose meant to quickly create an effective concentration of the medicine in your body. Two weeks later I had a second loading dose, and from there, a regular dose every other week to maintain the level of the drug. Like methotrexate, Humira is a subcutaneous injection (meaning applied under the skin, but not in a muscle), but instead of a needle and syringe, Humira comes preloaded in an injector, much like an EpiPen. I simply had to remove the pen from the box, clean a patch of skin on my thigh or abdomen with an alcohol swab, press the pen against my pinched skin and press the injector button.

It sounds simple enough, but the injection hurt like a bee sting and the medication burned like fire on the way in. I couldn't jerk my hand away because I needed every last drop of the medicine injected. It became increasingly harder to pull the trigger, anticipating the hot flash of pain to come. It would take fifteen minutes to work up the nerve, much like the feeling of standing on a high diving board trying to summon the courage to jump. Matt started injecting it for me, with a swift *1-2-3-click!* as I sat with my eyes squeezed shut, crushing his hand in mine at the stinging burn. The prick mark would be red and itchy for days afterward. Sometimes it was hard to find a spot to inject it that wasn't already red and irritated. (Interestingly, Humira is now available in a citrate-free formula that results in less discomfort at the injection site.)

I anticipate that she will eventually require removal of her remaining rectum with a permanent ileostomy, but she is reluctant to take that step at this time and will prefer to see how the disease responds to the Humira.

Those were the words in the follow-up report from my surgeon. That April, I had a consultation with him to discuss the recurring and persistent fistulas I'd been experiencing while on and off the methotrexate. We discussed my current treatment on Humira. While he expected I'd require further surgical intervention, he respected my desire to wait and see how well the Humira could control my disease.

The good news was that I responded to it well. I hadn't let Crohn's drag me down at this pivotal point in my life. My symptoms abated; I was thriving at my new gig as assistant editor at the lifestyle magazine; summer arrived—and with it, our wedding festivities.

Matt and I were the first of our friends to get married. My apartment with Christina became wedding-planning head-quarters. Both our boyfriends had condos nearby but, despite my recent engagement and pending nuptials, we chose to live together for one more year—our last chance to be the room-mates we'd always dreamed of, now that we were finally in the same city after four years apart at university. Our lease would come to an end shortly after the wedding. We'd slowly pack up the apartment and move on to the next chapter of our lives. Matt and I would move in together for the first time as a married couple.

If there was ever a "perfect" time to be healthy, this was it. Luck came my way, and I was symptom-free—no stomach pain, not even a cold sore, to which I was prone, especially in

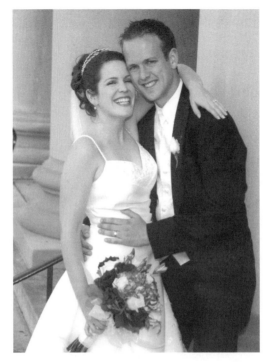

A lucky day! Heather's Crohn's symptoms were in remission on the day of her wedding to Matt Fegan, July 13, 2007.

times of stress. Even the thought of Crohn's was neatly packed away into a box and placed at the back of my mind.

A past fundraising campaign from what was then called the Crohn's and Colitis Foundation of Canada—now Crohn's and Colitis Canada—had depicted how IBD can show up unannounced at any time, how living with Crohn's means not knowing when you wake up each day whether you'll be fine or Crohn's will flare up and ruin your day, week, month, or even year. It was about never knowing whether you'll feel all right on your graduation or wedding day, or whether the vacation you've planned will be spoiled. The campaign featured a series of photos depicting these important milestones. I desperately did not want to become that poster child.

Fortunately, I managed to be well. I enjoyed my bridal shower, my bachelorette party out on the town, our rehearsal dinner—all the rites of passage for a new bride in the weeks leading up to our ceremony. We celebrated our nuptials with a big wedding with all our friends and family, a guest list of two hundred people. Matt's friends and relatives flew in from the UK, I had family from across Canada. Everyone important in our lives was together in that room. Two days later we left for a week-long honeymoon in Costa Rica without so much as a blip.

But of course, my Crohn's wouldn't let me get too comfortable as we settled into married life. The trial study I'd participated in had come to an end in September. I had done well, so we decided to continue the Humira injection every two weeks. Thankfully I had coverage for it on my drug plan because the cost for this kind of biologic treatment was astronomical, running anywhere from $21,000 to $36,000 per year for a standard dose—beyond anything I could afford out-of-pocket. The drug plan covered 80 percent of the cost and the remaining 20 percent was covered by a patient-support program through the drug manufacturer.

Come November, my Crohn's was starting to flare up in full force. Those big red and purple bumps, the erythema nodosum that I'd experienced years ago, returned on my legs. I had more than one fistula, some now escalated to abscesses on my backside. With my health declining, my doctor doubled my dose of Humira to gain control of my symptoms. In March 2008, my doctor decided to start from scratch. I was to restart with a high loading dose, followed by half that amount two weeks later and half of that amount two weeks after that. Then I would take a weekly dose of twice the amount I'd taken when I'd first started the drug. The reason for this "reintroduction" was that I had had such an excellent response when I'd first been introduced to Humira the year before; we wanted to hit my body with a high dose of it again. My symptoms improved and initially I did well. But when I had another scope that spring, it showed very active disease in my remaining bowel.

"We are using a lot of medication to treat a small area of severe disease," Dr. Farina said to me at an appointment that summer. "We should discuss the medical versus surgical options around your disease management."

It was a year into our marriage and Matt was now officially a part of my healthcare discussions. The small area of severe disease could be removed, but that would leave me with an ileostomy again. Though having children was nowhere on our radar at that point, it was part of our future plan. We wanted to avoid any more surgery due to the possible risk of infertility, so we struck that option off the table.

By October, I was no longer responding well to the Humira. I was on a high dose yet still experiencing a recurring flare and persistent symptoms. The disease was not progressing, nor was it in remission. I was in limbo, as when I had been on methotrexate, teetering on either side of acceptable baseline health and just getting by. I was getting a lot of canker sores in my mouth and now some abscess-like lesions were popping up on my inner thighs and along my groin—almost like ingrown hairs or folliculitis—that would spontaneously rupture. I'd also been having a lot of night sweats.

My doctor reassured me that we had given the biologic drug a good try. He said I'd likely need surgery; he wanted Matt and I to revisit the idea of a permanent ileostomy to remove what was left of the disease, diverting my ileum to my side once again. I was booked to consult with the surgeon at the end of the month, but in the meantime, my doctor prescribed another round of antibiotics to try and help clear up the mess. I went back on them—Cipro and Flagyl—and they worked. I'd love to say miraculously but it was purely scientific—the antibiotics kicked my system into high gear this time, in all the right ways. By the end of the month, in tandem with the Humira, the fistulas improved, my symptoms faded away, and there was no current indication of active Crohn's in the remaining bowel. At the follow-up consultation with my surgeon, because my symptoms had improved, the doctor noted: *Surgical intervention does not need to be discussed at this time.* I'd dodged another bullet.

MY FELLOW CROHNIE: JULIE'S JOURNEY

I met Julie Malone (she was a McCarthy back then, before she was married) during my first hospital admission, in grade 9. What were the chances I'd meet another girl my age, in my grade, with a similar disease, who was in the hospital at the same time? She had Crohn's disease, and at the time I had been diagnosed with ulcerative colitis, but we both had IBD. I was new to the whole thing, while Julie had a few years of experience—and some surgeries—under her belt.

Meeting Julie gave me the comfort of knowing I wasn't alone. There was someone just like me, going through the same thing. Julie lived in Hantsport, NS, and although we lived forty-five minutes apart, our parents helped us keep in touch over the years by driving us to one another's homes. Julie would visit me in the city, and I would go to the small town where she lived, where we would swim together in her pool. We went to conferences for teens with chronic illness. It was great to spend time with someone who could understand what I was going through, and to have someone to ask questions of shamelessly, especially while we were coming of age. We stayed in touch through high school, and though we pursued different programs on different campuses in university, we partied together and went out to eat occasionally. Over the years we've popped into one another's inboxes with occasional questions and check-ins—sometimes years apart, but that never matters. I attended her wedding, though she couldn't make it to mine. She was pregnant before me, and I was able to gain some insight into her experience to help make my own decisions. What a comfort it has been, knowing I wasn't alone.

This is the story of Julie's journey with Crohn's disease.

Julie's symptoms began when she was twelve years old. Her illness started with abdominal pain, diarrhea, and weight fluctuations. "It was kind of insidious in the way it slowly worked its way into my life," she says. "I'd be sick for three or four weeks and then it would go away. It would never stay long enough to really pursue it."

One summer, her grandmother came to visit. She took one look at Julie and told Julie's mom: "You need to get that girl checked out."

"I was skin and bones and I'd never been a super-thin child; I was always kind of curvy," says Julie. "At that point I had an ultrasound and they sent me very quickly, within a week, to the IWK. At that time they were using indium scans to diagnose Crohn's. My mom recalls sitting there and looking at the scan and seeing it glow like a Christmas tree, and just having a sinking feeling roll over her while I lay there, oblivious, on the table. She realized it was inflammation. I was sent up to Dr. Ste-Marie that day and was diagnosed with Crohn's."

With very few treatment options available for young people, the initial treatment for Julie's Crohn's was tube feeding. Julie started on enteral feedings twenty hours a day. "The challenge was that the system was really poorly set up, so I remember having a big vest of feeds on my chest, which is not very cool when you're a teen—walking around with this big bulky pack and a tube in your nose, in junior high."

The feeding tube made life difficult for the young teenager, and it wasn't really helping with her Crohn's.

"Early on I put on some weight and grew a few inches, so that

Tube feeding (enteral feeding) is necessary when a person can't take food in by mouth; nutrition is delivered via a flexible tube inserted either through the nose or directly into the stomach or small intestine.

was good. But I wasn't getting better in the sense that I was still having a lot of abdominal pain; [I was] still really sick," says Julie.

A year later she was still having severe pain and was admitted to hospital. Her care team cycled her through various medications. Then they made a shocking discovery—pills she had taken weeks ago were still undigested. Her bowel was so rock-hard the pills could not break down or move through.

Julie needed her first surgery at the age of thirteen to remove that foot and a half of bowel. Still, she didn't get better. After bouncing in and out of hospital for six months, doctors discovered they'd cut off the supply of blood to her nerves, and she had a second surgery to remove another chunk of bowel. Rounds of TPN followed.

That year, Julie was present for only sixty-eight days of her grade 9 school year; she was absent for sixty-nine. Yet she still graduated as an honours student, with an average in the high eighties.

"I always really pushed to make sure I did well at school," says Julie. "I think I missed the first six weeks of [grade 10] because I was in hospital and I still scored really high, because it…was the one thing I had. I couldn't do sports; I wasn't well enough. I didn't feel super pretty; I had that moon face. So school was the thing I really held on to."

Life carried on for Julie, with recurrent admissions to hospital.

"I think a few times [the doctors] started thinking it was like Munchausen by proxy or even my own Munchausen,"

Munchausen syndrome is a mental health disorder in which a person pretends to have a physical or mental illness. Munchausen by proxy is a similar disorder in which a caregiver falsifies an illness for someone in their care.

Julie says, laughing at the absurdity of the idea that she or her parents would pretend she was ill, "because they really struggled sometimes to find the reasons I'd be having so much pain or I wouldn't gain weight. The diagnostic tests and the treatments were so limited that they were getting frustrated." Even azathioprine (Imuran), a common treatment now for early-stage Crohn's that helps to reduce inflammation in the intestines, could only be administered off-label with permission from a Health Canada Special Access Program, as the drug wasn't approved for pediatric use, or to treat Crohn's disease back then. Julie's mother had to wear gloves just to dole it out because of its toxicity.

"There was so little known, no biologics on the market back then," says Julie. "It was prednisone or tube-feeds or surgery." Julie was allergic to many of the 5-ASA drugs, which never worked for her anyway, so they weren't a treatment option.

One of the few bright spots from her illness was that it gave her the opportunity to go on a Sunshine DreamLift, an experience funded by the Sunshine Foundation of Canada in which an airplane full of sick kids and youth are flown to a Disney theme park and back home in just one day.

"It was a pretty interesting time in my life, going between school and the hospital," says Julie. "That was most of my junior high years. In high school, I did okay. There were probably a few periods where I was quite sick, but I was on prednisone. I think that was really the hard part of high school—having the big moon face as a teenager, and the hormones, and not murdering my mother and her not murdering me back," Julie laughs. Along with headaches, dizziness, and trouble sleeping, other side effects of prednisone include acne, chubby cheeks—moon face—and extreme mood swings. "It was not feeling attractive, and all that stuff that goes with that period of your life [was] intensified with steroids. I think that was very formative in [terms of] my self-image later in life." Julie had to have more tube-feeds to give her energy and the ability to function, but she chose to put the tube in and take it out by herself each day, rather than wear it twenty-four hours a day.

Then came university. And dorms. And having Crohn's while living in a communal area, having diarrhea all the time. Within six weeks, she developed her first abscess, along with a recto-vaginal fistula that brutally persisted until recent years. "It was really interesting, starting to navigate a sex life and having this fistula," says Julie. "It was kind of an awkward phase of developing as a woman but having this disability."

Julie was happy to graduate from the children's hospital, where a healthcare provider had once told her there was nothing more they could offer her. She loved her new gastroenterologist, Dr. Kareemi. "He was fabulous," says Julie. "I just adored him. He was always really supportive and helpful."

But Julie was never able to find true remission. She tried Remicade a few times when it was new to the market, but it was expensive. With Julie in university, her family couldn't afford it. After three treatments that did not make a significant difference, she stopped the medication. She navigated life with the illness, taking prednisone here and there as needed.

Then, at age nineteen, a life-threatening infection nearly killed her. After having her wisdom teeth removed, Julie was rushed to the hospital in Halifax on Christmas Day with a heart murmur, extremely high liver enzymes, and a high white blood-cell count. She was admitted to hospital and put on IV antibiotics for a week.

"You don't think of the comorbidities of having a chronic illness," says Julie. "The thing that almost kills you isn't necessarily the disease but the immunosuppression [caused by] treating the disease," explains Julie. "That was my one big brush with death."

Julie recovered and went on to graduate from the Respiratory Therapy program at the School of Health Sciences at Dalhousie University. She started working right away, landing a job at The Moncton Hospital in New Brunswick. Her Crohn's was somewhat in check, but she cycled through drugs, taking methotrexate (an immune-system suppressant) and azathioprine, her treatments always very transient. Something would work for a year, then stop. She'd resort back to steroids for a while and then try a different immunosuppressive for a period of time. That one would stop working, so back on the steroids she'd go.

Julie started doing drug trials to find something—anything—that would help her. She finally found a drug that worked; it was a treatment often used for multiple sclerosis. But in the MS population it was being mixed with another immunosuppressive that was causing a dangerous ALS-type syndrome so the drug was yanked off the market. The treatment was no longer available for her. (ALS—Amyotrophic lateral sclerosis, also known as Lou Gehrig's disease, is a neurological disease that affects the nerve cells in the brain and spinal cord that control voluntary muscle movement.)

"That was the first time I finally almost went into full remission, and I'd just gotten permission for two years of the drug covered by the drug company, and I was so upset because that was the first time I felt really, really good," says Julie. "Within six months I was back in hospital."

A year and a half into starting her career, Julie's health crashed; she lost thirty pounds very quickly and landed in hospital for over a month. "I was dating different people, so no one really noticed," she says. Even the nurse practitioner she was seeing hadn't picked up on how bad things were.

For a while after that admission, Julie's health stabilized. She went back on Remicade, a biologic that helped for a couple of years, then switched to another new biologic, Humira, for a couple of years. She met the man who would later become her husband, and they packed up and moved to Toronto in 2007. Julie landed one of the leading physicians in the country, Dr. Hillary Steinhart, as her GI specialist. "I think my referral was specifically to him for a reason because I am so complex and not an easy Crohn's, but he took me on. He called me a 'severe, aggressive, complex Crohn's patient.'"

Julie got married in 2008, and a year later, not knowing if it was going to be easy or not, got pregnant. "The more abdominal surgeries you have, it reduces your fertility a lot, but we got pregnant right away."

Julie had to stop working when she was twenty-four weeks pregnant due to a flare-up. She received a double dose of Remicade to try to get things under control—and wound up with shingles. Although she was very ill throughout her pregnancy, in February 2010, at thirty-seven weeks and four days, she gave birth to a healthy baby boy who weighed eight pounds, four ounces. Julie says she considers herself very fortunate, though it took her years to recover. "That's a big reason we only have one," she says. "It sucked every bit of good out of me and I just never really felt well again." She continued to fight to find something that would help her, struggling through rounds of methotrexate, Remicade, and steroids.

By this point, Julie had been doing shift work for years, and she was beginning to get worn out despite her good intentions. "I wanted to help people and I [had been] impacted by the people in my life who worked in health care. I think [my illness] made me a really empathetic, caring person, [able] to understand those going through a health crisis," she says. But respiratory therapists are routinely exposed to and susceptible to viruses and infections. "It may not have been the wisest career choice," she acknowledges, "so I started to look into [getting] a Monday to Friday job that didn't involve night shifts."

Julie took courses through her employment at Toronto General Hospital, and by 2015 she made the move to a leadership role. "As a manager in health care, when people don't meet the needs of patients, it pushes me harder to make sure my team knows the expectations and what they need to do. I set those expectations very clearly because I think it's really important, having gone through the other side of it."

She limped along with her own health until a new drug called Entyvio (vedolizumab) came on the market. Julie was one of the first patients, if not *the* first patient in Canada, to take it. It had been released to treat ulcerative colitis, but it was the first treatment to ever put her into remission. She became well enough to be considered for surgery to have her still-persistent fistula fixed. At that point her fistula was so bad it leaked gas and stool, which made daily life difficult.

"It was horrific," says Julie. "I think of all the things that went on in my life—surgery, TPN, and tube feedings—and this was probably the most debilitating part of my life." With her Crohn's at the best it had ever been, she says it was a strike-now-or-never type of situation. Julie would need a temporary ileostomy to divert her remaining bowel away from the fistula site to allow things to heal.

It took months and months to get in to see a surgeon, and months and months on a wait-list after that. During this period, her sister was diagnosed with cancer: appendiceal adenocarcinoma.

"I got my surgery date...[and] on the same day my sister got told her cancer had moved from stage three to stage four," says Julie. "I found out my surgery was in a week. It was very rough timing, family-wise, trying to figure it out with a kid and living in Toronto on our own." Julie and her husband both worked very busy jobs, and they weren't sure how they were going to manage the to-and-from school. "That was a challenge," says Julie. "My mom came up but then felt this guilt of trying to be in two places at once. How do you manage that with one daughter fighting for her life and the other having chunks of her bowel cut out and dealing with having an ostomy for the first time?" Julie says family on both sides pitched in to help and make sure her son Jonah was taken care of. "It was a wild time."

But after the surgery in February 2018, Julie didn't feel better. Nonetheless, she returned to work. "I think it has a lot to do with having been chronically ill but really always being stubborn and being like, 'I'm not sick.'" She was, in fact, so unwell she could barely walk. Finally, one evening after work, she got off her bus and wasn't sure she could make it the five hundred feet to her front door. "That was scary because it was a busy road and I could've been hit by a car," she says.

She called her doctor, who instructed her to get blood work. He phoned soon after to tell her that her creatine was so high she was in renal failure. She was admitted to hospital for treatment for a month—a typical stay for her. "I had to laugh because my sister and I were both laying in Emerg because she had gotten sick too, and we were sending each other 'who wore it better' selfies in our hospital gowns. You get kind of sick and twisted."

During her hospital stay, tests showed the fistula repair hadn't worked, so she went back on the wait-list—four and a half months long—for more surgery.

Eventually Julie was able to go home with a PICC line and an IV pump so she could self-treat with fluids every night to heal her renal failure. She'd head off to work on the subway with the PICC line hanging out of her arm, but often had to stand on the train and watch others take the seats reserved for people with disabilities. "I was so bitter," she admits. "I tried not to judge because Crohn's is an invisible illness, so maybe they [too] had a condition you couldn't see. But…I think they were probably just jerks."

Julie came to terms with the fact that after twenty years, there was no fixing her fistula. She decided it wasn't worth it to her to keep trying. "It was too much time off work, too much time away from my family, too much risk," says Julie. "So on October 25, 2018, I had my ileostomy reversed and a permanent colostomy done." A proctectomy—surgery to remove all of her rectum, including the fistula—was done laparoscopically, but the time and positioning on the operating room table left her with a debilitating back injury that led to four months of physio.

A peripherally inserted central catheter (PICC) is a tube that is inserted into a vein that is used on a long-term basis to give intravenous fluids, blood transfusions, chemotherapy, and other drugs.

Julie worked through the physio and got used to her permanent ostomy. Now she's working to get her life back. "I never eat really well," she says. "There's always that psychological difficulty with food. You eat something, it hurts, you don't eat it anymore. I think we all have some form of disordered eating that we develop over the years with our Crohn's. I can't even think of fibre; it scares me. I still get pain from a lot of fibre. But I love my carbs." Julie jokes that gluten is her main food staple, along with potato chips, and admits to struggling to get proper nutrition, which affects her ability to encourage her son to eat healthy foods by example.

She worries about the effect her illness has had on her son. "Being in the hospital for his birthday—it has a significant impact on him." When he was very young, she could rest while he was napping, but now her downtimes are harder to disguise. "[If] I'm feeling unwell when I get home, he'll give me a big hug because he can tell I'm just exhausted. He's a wonderfully empathetic kid, and probably me being sick has a bit to do with [him] developing those skills. Then you have that intense mom-guilt."

On a day-to-day level, living with Crohn's can be a grind. "I try to balance doing what I can when I can do it," she explains. "You learn that early on; you do what you can when you can do it because you don't know when the next thing is going to come around the corner. I'm worse this week than I was [in] the two weeks before this."

Julie took advantage of feeling well in 2019 to complete a master of arts in leadership, and eventually relocated with her family back to Nova Scotia for a Health Services manager role with the Nova Scotia Health Authority. "A year later I might not have felt well enough, so you try to find those points when life lets you go there." The days when she doesn't want to get out of bed can be tough. "Everyone else is trying to be your cheerleader and you're like, 'Not today. I'm going to lay in bed in pain and I just want my hot water bottle and to eat chips and I want you all to leave me alone.'"

When we spoke, Julie thought she might be flaring up, but says Crohn's affects her less now than it used to. Before her last surgery she had to really think about things like where the bathrooms were at work and which of those were private, or whether to go out for a meal if she didn't know where the bathroom was or whether she could make it home on the subway. Now, with an ostomy, she's much more free—able to do things like camp and travel without worrying.

"I do everything now," she says. "I'm way less restricted. Going to the beach and wearing a bikini—I still do it. If someone doesn't like the look of it, who cares? I love that high-waisted bikinis are in. They are way easier than other two-piece bathing suits and you can't see my ostomy."

She does admit those things would have been harder when she was younger.

"People need to know it's not so shameful," says Julie. "It's come a long way. We're seeing underwear commercials with ostomies in them. I think it's great."

She says women with Crohn's tend to be strong. "I've met some badass women over the years; one's a CEO of a foundation. You can accomplish a lot having a diagnosis of Crohn's," she says. "I didn't do too badly [in life], considering I have a very severe form of a nasty chronic autoimmune disease. I could have tapped out long ago and I decided not to."

She turns to me. "You and I spent a lot of time in the hospital and we've both done pretty well. We have careers; families; we've gotten married. Young girls need to know that. If we [had] met women like us when we were teens, imagine…," Julie trails off.

We didn't know what the future held, but meeting someone just like me when I was a teen helped. Julie was someone I could connect with, relate to, and feel inspired by. We didn't focus on it at the time, but I understand now it made all the difference in the world to know I wasn't alone.

Julie and I are proof that people with Crohn's disease can live a great life. We can do anything anyone else can do—maybe even more. Our tolerance for pain is high. We're used to pushing through when we're not feeling 100 percent. Crohn's comes with a lot, including incredible strength and the determination to keep on going. Crohn's creates warriors.

"I'm a person and I live with Crohn's," says Julie. "I have Crohn's, but it doesn't have me. ...I live with it, it affects me, and I make some accommodations in my life for it, but I'm not my disease. ...That's no way to live."

There are plenty of famous people with IBD who don't let their disease hold them back:

- Kathleen Baker, American Olympic swimmer
- Pete Davidson, actor, writer (*Saturday Night Live*, *The King of Staten Island*)
- Jake Diekman, Major League Baseball player (Tampa Bay Rays)
- Shannen Doherty, actress (*Beverly Hills, 90210*)
- Jimmy Donaldson, aka MrBeast, YouTuber
- Darren Fletcher, former English Premier League soccer player
- Ashley Freeborn, Founder and CEO of Smash + Tess clothing label
- David Garrard, former NFL football player

- Hank Green, YouTuber and author (*An Absolutely Remarkable Thing*)
- Carrie Johnson, American Olympic kayaker
- Matt Light, former NFL football player
- Chuck Lorre, producer and director (*Big Bang Theory*, *Two and a Half Men*)
- Mike McCready, lead guitarist, Pearl Jam
- Audra McDonald, Tony award-winning Broadway performer
- Larry Nance Jr., NBA basketball player (New Orleans Pelicans)
- Dan O'Bannon, screenwriter and director (*The Return of the Living Dead*, *The Resurrected*)
- Sir Steve Redgrave, British Olympic rower
- Dan Reynolds, lead vocalist, Imagine Dragons
- Tyler James Williams, Golden Globe–winning actor (*Abbott Elementary*)

MY STORY:
ADVENTURES WITH
REMICADE

(2008–2012)

With my Crohn's mostly in remission, it wasn't long before I developed something new to contend with—something called hidradenitis suppurativa (HS). It's a painful, long-term skin condition that causes abscesses and scarring on the skin. The exact cause of hidradenitis suppurativa is unknown, but it occurs near hair follicles where there are sweat glands, and for me this was around my groin and inner thighs. It had started flaring up that fall when the antibiotics had done the trick to get me into remission. Hidradenitis and Crohn's are separate entities, but they do coexist in about 1 percent of Crohn's patients—lucky me. I was referred to a dermatologist for treatment, but hidradenitis is difficult to treat.

The dermatologist recommended that we consider switching to Remicade, as there was some case literature to indicate that it is a beneficial treatment for this skin problem. Remicade is similar to Humira, in that it's also a biologic immunosuppressive drug that helps stop inflammation by blocking TNF–α.

Over the next few months there was a lot of discussion around the risks and benefits of me switching to Remicade.

There was no way to know if it would help, but all we could do was try. If it didn't work, I could switch back to Humira. In the meantime, my Crohn's seemed to be bubbling under the surface, nagging at me in the background while I pressed on with life.

Dr. Farina was not actually 100 percent happy with my results with Humira anyway. He told me I downplayed my symptoms, even when I said I felt good. Since I was not actually in optimal health, he suggested at least trying Remicade to see if it helped more than the Humira. Remicade is effective for both fistulizing Crohn's and hidradenitis, so it was worth a shot since I was experiencing those very symptoms. He recommended trying three doses to see how I would respond.

The challenge was that I was covered for the cost of Humira on a small private drug plan, and I was already pushing its limits; I wasn't sure I could get the same coverage for Remicade, which was equally expensive. My doctor asked me to look into my drug coverage—a long and complicated process that took a long time to coordinate.

In the meantime, I carried on with Humira. The drug had to be kept refrigerated but I didn't let that tie me down. In the spring, Matt and I took a holiday to Ireland. I toted the medication along with me in a lunch bag with freezer packs. I asked the flight attendants to keep it cold on the flight. On our first night, I asked reception at the hotel to keep it in the fridge in the kitchen since our room didn't have a mini-fridge. The next day we were about a thirty-minute drive away from the hotel, on the way to our next stop, when I remembered where the drug was. We had to circle back to collect it. I was then able to keep it in the fridge at our next destination, my sister-in-law's place, until it was time to inject it. Then we were back home before it was time for my next dose. It took a little extra coordination to travel with the drug, but it was certainly worth it.

Finally, a few months later, with the assistance of a nurse coordinator, I was awarded exceptional drug coverage status to assist with the cost of the new medication. In June 2009 it was finally time to start Remicade. As with Humira, there was a loading process. Remicade is given by intravenous (IV) infusion, rather than being injected with a needle. I received my first infusion at week zero, my second at two weeks, and a third dose at six weeks. The standard would then be an infusion every eight weeks. I received these infusions at a private clinic, conveniently located across the street from my office. I had a new job, as the managing editor of a magazine about books and publishing. The lifestyle publication had folded and I had seamlessly switched to this new job. The office was small—just me and a co-worker. It was quiet, but very busy, managing marketing and communications for an association of book publishers. On the day of my infusion, I'd gather up files and papers, head across the street, and work away while the medication dripped into my veins, working its magic.

The treatment typically takes a couple of hours to infuse. The clinic was small and basic and felt like a waiting room, but instead of uncomfortable straight-backed chairs there were four or five oversized brown recliners in a row, each holding a patient hooked up to an IV pump that whirred away and occasionally beeped. The clinic was run by nurses who got the IV lines going then bustled around, filling out paperwork at their desks, chatting with patients, and checking vitals every thirty minutes to make sure everyone was stable. The nurses monitored the infusion speed, adjusting the rate at which the medication was administered—slowly at first, increasing in speed as the appointment went on. This was to make sure the body could tolerate the medication and that it could be infused without causing issues or reactions.

At every other appointment, as my IV was inserted the nurses would draw blood to be sent off to the lab for screening, looking for any abnormal results. Once the IV line was running, it was hurry up and wait. There was a TV in the clinic, which I never paid much attention to as I tried to get my work done, tuning out whatever had been chosen by whoever had gotten their hands on the remote first. The nurses offered up snacks, coffee and tea, and cozy blankets. Once my appointment was over, I'd head back to my office.

After my third dose of Remicade, I was feeling a lot better. I had more energy and was feeling much improved, Crohn's-wise. I noticed a slight improvement with the hidradenitis. Rather than wait six or eight weeks for my first regular dose, my doctor decided to give it after four weeks in hope of seeing even more improvement. Figuring out the best schedule of treatment was going to be a game of wait-and-see. In a note to my family doctor, Dr. Farina said:

> [Regarding] the subsequent maintenance dose, I think we are simply going to have to determine her schedule. She has required a higher dose of Humira than normal and, therefore, she may not simply achieve maintenance with q.8* weeks. I have sent her for an additional break-through dose this time and will schedule her for q.8 weeks after that. However, I will make any adjustments based on symptoms and if they return at an earlier date, we will certainly get her in earlier.

> *(*Ed's note: "q." is shorthand for "each" or "every.")*

My infusion in October 2009 fell on my birthday. I thought it was a wise move to schedule my appointment that day to allow for a more relaxing afternoon with my feet up, but after half an hour of the infusion, I developed a fever. My temperature jumped from thirty-six to thirty-eight and continued to rise. The nurse immediately slowed the infusion down, pushed Benadryl through my IV, and gave me Tylenol. My temperature slowly returned to normal, and I was able to gradually finish the infusion. It took an extra two hours, and I almost missed my birthday dinner. I made it, although I was groggy from the extra medication.

After following up with my doctor, it was decided that the clinic would need to administer Benadryl and Tylenol at every infusion moving forward. Unfortunately, that wouldn't be my last reaction.

November 12, 2009
Patient Name: Fegan, Heather
Report sent to: Dr. David T. MacNeil, family physician

Dear Dr. MacNeil:

I reviewed Heather in the clinic today. She is a very pleasant 27-year-old female, who I have been following for quite some time for Crohn's disease. She also has quite significant HS. For this she has been seeing Dr. Green. In regard to her symptoms, she is doing quite well on Remicade. She does have a good symptom response for the first 4-6 weeks; however, after six weeks her symptoms seem to deteriorate. At this point, I think we should put her on a more frequent dosing, between 4-6 weeks of Remicade. She wants to try a 6-week interval as it is quite expensive and causing quite a significant burden on her drug plan. Therefore, we will try her on a 6-week interval and re-evaluate her in three months' time with the view of seeing how she is doing clinically.

Yours sincerely,
Dana M. Farina, MD, FRCPC
Attending Staff, Dept. of Med (Gastroenterology)

Sure enough, eight weeks between doses was too long. I'd feel great after my infusion, and at some point between six and eight weeks later, symptoms would start to flare. This little song and dance of moving around my treatment times carried on over the next several months. A flare-up in February 2010 had me needing a dose after just four weeks. Then I was scheduled to have the medication regularly at five-week intervals, despite my health plan giving me trouble for increasing the frequency of such an expensive drug. We fought back, and I remained on the drug plan.

By April, I needed another dose four weeks after my last. My routine blood work showed low hemoglobin. I was anemic, so I was prescribed weekly iron infusions for five weeks. My symptoms were flaring up even as I reached the four-week interval. My doctor said it was time to reassess the disease.

It was summer before I could get a scope, which showed:

> ...multiple fistulas. The remaining bowel was diffusely inflamed and thickened over a few centimetres. The anastomosis has some mild erosions at the anastomosis however the subsequent 20 to 30 centimetres of the bowel was completely normal. Overall, the findings today are significant Crohn's in a very short segment. At this point I think our best option would be to do a diversion ileostomy however I think it would be important for Heather to contemplate these options a bit more. I will see her again in follow-up.

Despite the poor results and another call for surgery, I managed to rebound again. I was a human yoyo, bouncing between sickness and health. This was the kicker with my Crohn's: every time it seemed like another surgery was imminent, I'd get a small window of improvement—enough for me to push through, thinking I was healthy (or healthy enough).

But that's the thing with a chronic illness. It will not stay away forever. Somehow by August I improved enough to tag along on Matt's work trip to Paris so we could pop over to his cousin's wedding in England while we were there (thanks again to British discount airlines). We created nothing but great memories on the trip; Crohn's did not slow me down. Still, there was no rhyme or reason to it. I did nothing differently. The truth was, sometimes my body worked for me and sometimes it worked against me.

December 14, 2010
Patient Name: Fegan, Heather
Report sent to: Dr. David T. MacNeil, family physician

Dear Dr. MacNeil:

I reviewed Heather in the clinic today. She is a very pleasant 28-year-old female who I have been following for Crohn's disease. At present she is doing reasonably well on Remicade q.4 weeks. She does have intermittent episodes where she will have increasing symptoms prior to her infusion. At this point, we have had discussions with Heather again that she is on a relatively high dose of Remicade for a fairly short segment of disease. We have again discussed surgical options with her. She is certainly comfortable with her current management and wishes to continue on the current course. I will see her again in four months' time and keep you informed of our findings.

Yours sincerely,
Dana M. Farina, MD, FRCPC
Attending Staff, Dept. of Med (Gastroenterology)

When I was seen at the clinic in December 2010—pleasant, as always, despite my plight—my doctor and I discussed the findings in that report. Yes, I was on a relatively high dose of Remicade for a fairly small area of disease within my digestive system, but knowing the alternative—surgery and a permanent ileostomy and the risk of infertility that could come with it—I decided I was comfortable with the current management of my Crohn's and stayed the course—the extremely rocky course. And so it went, with my infusion every four weeks. Sometimes I'd flare up right before my treatment, then I'd respond well to the treatment, but that good response would wane over the next four weeks. In March 2011, a particularly bad flare landed me in the emergency department with fever and chills—there was an infection somewhere in the mess of fistulas and abscesses and I was put back on antibiotics. Dr. Farina once again gently nudged me to consider the surgical side of disease management. He set up a consultation with a new surgeon—mine had since retired—but I cancelled the appointment. Throughout it all, I didn't miss a beat. I summoned the strength to continue to enjoy my life as I believed it should be enjoyed, just as everyone else I knew did. I stood in friends' weddings, took holidays, and worked hard at my job.

August 30, 2011
Patient Name: Fegan, Heather
Report sent to: Dr. Elena Swift, family physician

Dear Elena:

I reviewed Heather in the clinic today. She is a very pleasant 28-year-old female who I have been following for inflammatory bowel disease....
    [She] and her husband are still in the process of contemplating pregnancy. I think given her active

perianal disease at present, it would be best to get it under better control. In regard to this, I am going to add Cipro to her medication as she does get good response from this...I do feel that she should also speak to the surgeon. I had set up an appointment... in the past, however, she cancelled it. She does have a very short segment of disease, which is causing quite a significant problem and is slowly losing response to Remicade.

In regard to other issues, I think it would be reasonable to have her seen by the maternal fetal medicine physician in terms of pre-pregnancy counselling.

I will make those arrangements and keep you informed of our findings.

Yours sincerely,
Dana M. Farina, MD, FRCPC
Attending Staff, Dept. of Med (Gastroenterology)

I was having another bad flare in August when I had a follow-up appointment in the GI clinic. Once again, my pleasant demeanor was noted in the report back to my family physician, this time to the new family doctor I'd started seeing in the same family practice. No matter how sick I am, at least I'm always pleasant to my doctors! I was continuing to experience episodes where my symptoms would increase and I would develop a fever during the week prior to the Remicade infusion.

At that point there was not much more for my doctor to offer me besides antibiotics, which always seemed to help just enough to keep me going. While having kids was part of our plan, we weren't quite ready yet, although we knew it was something we would have to plan for well in advance to be sure I was in optimal health—hence the referral for pre-pregnancy counselling.

In October, my symptoms took a turn. I was having sharp pains in my abdomen and feeling really bloated; my trips to the bathroom were less frequent. I booked an urgent appointment at the GI clinic and saw a nurse practitioner who advised me to go to the emergency department to be assessed. My own GI doctor, Dr. Farina, happened to be on call—a blessing, as he knew my history. An abdominal X-ray showed distended loops of air-filled bowel. I had a partial bowel obstruction which meant I couldn't go home.

When the doctor told me I was being admitted, I burst into tears. There was a look of confusion on Dr. Farina's face as he cautiously asked what was wrong. What was wrong?! I was in pain. I was exhausted. I was disappointed. Crohn's had just scored a point in our battle, knocking me down and into a hospital bed, a place I hadn't been since surgery. The constant teetering on the edge between sickness and health was completely draining and I was swaying in the wrong direction.

"I'm supposed to go apple-picking with my friends tomorrow!" I blubbered through my tears. I understood my doctor's look of confusion. The show of emotion was out of the ordinary for me—I was known for my poker face. I hadn't shed a tear over Crohn's since the day I'd been confronted with the decision to have the first surgery and I'd dropped into Matt's arms in tears. But by this point I'd been through so much for so long that, despite my strength, my mask had slipped. Missing the apple picking trip wasn't actually a big deal. I angrily swiped the tears away. "Sorry. It's just a lot."

He gave my arm a pat as he left the room. "You'll be okay."

On top of everything, it was Thanksgiving weekend—a weekend made for eating—and I had been admitted to hospital on bowel rest, meaning no food or drink allowed. It also meant I would miss out on quality time with friends and family.

It was an uneventful hospital stay. Matt hung out with me during the day and we mostly watched TV. I was put on IV fluids and treated with methylprednisolone (Solu-Medrol), a synthetic corticosteroid delivered via IV, and antibiotics. The pain settled and very soon I was feeling better. A second set of X-rays showed less distension right away. Things were improving and I was able to ease back onto a soft diet with no problems. I switched to oral prednisone and four days later I was allowed to go home, with an appointment to see a surgeon already booked.

On October 20, 2011, I met with my new colorectal surgeon to discuss the possibility of surgery to manage my Crohn's disease. I was feeling well from the treatment of the bowel obstruction, but I could hardly cancel the appointment again, given my recent hospital admission. I had it in my mind that I needed to be off Remicade before getting pregnant; if I went off the medication, surgery was the alternative treatment.

When I met with the surgeon to discuss this option, he ordered two tests—a small bowel follow-through (a form of real-time x-ray that produces images of the small intestine) and a flexible sigmoidoscopy—to rule out proximal Crohn's disease. If there was no sign of Crohn's disease beyond the area we already knew about, I'd be a very good candidate for a diverting ileostomy. I knew this, but really wasn't interested in pursuing a surgical option. This was both to protect my fertility and because I simply did not want an ileostomy again. The surgeon said we'd plan to avoid any pelvic surgery (not removing the rectum, just diverting the ileum through the side of my abdomen) until after any pregnancies due to the greater risk of infertility with that procedure. He explained that there was already some risk of infertility as a result of prior inflammation and previous surgeries, but hopefully that risk was not very high. We'd meet again to discuss the findings. Neither Matt nor I wanted to have to consider these surgical options, even one with the lowest risk of affecting my fertility, but we also needed to find a way for me to have a healthy pregnancy. We decided we'd cross that bridge if—or when—we got to it.

Less than a month later, on a drab, grey day in November, Matt and I sat in a stark clinical exam room at the IWK Health Centre, which also has a women's and newborn health service. We had been referred through the Perinatal Centre to the Preconception Counselling Clinic for advice surrounding pregnancy and my health. We went through my entire history— medical, social, family, gynecological—with a resident who took detailed notes. Then we went over my current medications—Remicade and Cipro; I had just finished the steroids prescribed during my hospital admission.

When the resident finished his questions, he left for a bit, returning with Dr. Michiel Van den Hof, a senior OB/GYN and maternal fetal medicine specialist. He guided us through an assessment in anticipation of a future pregnancy. We discussed the risks of a pregnancy complicated by Crohn's disease and the effect of pregnancy on the disease, as well as the importance of having the disease under optimal control at the time of conception (and in the three to six months before that). We discussed maternal and fetal risks associated with a Crohn's pregnancy—increased risk of preterm birth, intrauterine growth restriction, miscarriage, and fetal loss. These risks are much higher with poorly controlled disease. We discussed the mode of delivery, which, in the presence of severe disease, would have to be Caesarean section.

We also discussed medication use in pregnancy, with the doctor stressing the importance of appropriately controlled Crohn's disease, which I took to mean "Don't mess around with your treatments once you're pregnant because that could make things worse." He explained that Remicade had been used during pregnancies, though experience was limited. Researchers can't put pregnant women through trials with these drugs, but they can follow pregnancies during which the medication is used. There had been no congenital anomalies associated with Remicade, and he said he'd recommend continuing it during pregnancy if necessary. My ears perked up on hearing this. This was encouraging advice; I hadn't considered being able to continue my current course of treatment. He said that in the event of a flare-up, steroid therapy would be appropriate and well tolerated during pregnancy, though it does have an associated risk of gestational diabetes and fetal growth restriction.

Finally, we discussed how we would manage a potential Crohn's flare during pregnancy. The plan included an early ultrasound for determining the due date as well as an early pregnancy review and serum screening for genetic abnormalities. The amount of surveillance necessary would depend on how active my Crohn's disease was. If things were flaring up, ultrasounds for fetal growth and well-being would be done during the second and third trimesters, as they would for any pregnancies while I was on Remicade or steroids. I'd have a detailed ultrasound around twenty weeks' gestation to make sure everything was all right. I felt hopeful with all this information. I had full confidence in Dr. Van den Hof, what with his credentials.

Dr. Van den Hof wrapped up the appointment by saying he would be happy to see me and follow my pregnancy through the maternal fetal medicine clinic as well as the Fetal Assessment and Treatment Centre in the event I got pregnant. Matt and I felt optimistic leaving the clinic. The doctor would be happy to follow me in the event of a pregnancy! This was a much better outcome than advising against getting pregnant at all—a prognosis I'd feared hearing.

It came time for the scope, this one a rigid sigmoidoscopy. It wouldn't be too invasive, I was assured, and would be done without sedation, much to my dismay. The surgeon took one look into my rectum and, due to the strictures and severe scarring of the area, would not even proceed with the scope. He abruptly declared aloud that the short-term plan had to be surgery and that I absolutely needed a diverting stoma. I remained stone-cold silent. That was the end of the exam.

I was completely taken aback by the bluntness of this surgeon—his lack of empathy. In fact, I was furious. He might be fine with the idea of cutting me up, but I certainly wasn't. How could I go through with the surgery at a point when I was feeling well? ("Well" by my own—albeit skewed—standards.) I kept my cool until I had changed out of my johnny shirt and reunited with Matt in the waiting room. Then I unleashed angry tears, storming my way out of the hospital, ranting about the brusque, abrupt surgeon, Matt trailing behind me in confusion. I not only disagreed with the surgeon, I disliked him all together.

The small bowel follow-through was scheduled for a week later. I wasn't too concerned. I'd never presented evidence of Crohn's in my small intestine, but it was worth investigating in order to be sure. I swallowed barium, a chalky powder mixed with water that appears white on X-ray film, while they followed it down my gastrointestinal tract. The test showed no disease in my small bowel.

In the weeks that followed I continued to feel well, which left me on the fence about surgery. Maybe I didn't have to trade my meds in for an ileostomy. For the first time in a while, things felt somewhat under control. The medical team at the IWK had given me the go-ahead to get pregnant on my current treatment regime. By the time my next follow-up appointment came around at the GI clinic at the end of January 2012, I'd been off antibiotics for a month with no adverse effects. I decided I was no longer interested in pursuing a surgical option and was instead interested in starting to think about family planning. (Looking back, I can't help but feel justified in my frustration at the surgeon who so bluntly declared my imminent need for surgery. I guess he didn't realize he was up against a fighter. I requested to not be referred to him again.)

My GI doctor believed the best bet, at that point, was to completely optimize my medications. It had been a decade since I'd last been on azathioprine, which had elevated my liver enzymes. But there was another form of this drug called 6-MP, or mercaptopurine, which could be more easily tolerated. Dr. Farina didn't think it was unreasonable to try this medication. He thought the combination therapy would be much more likely to keep things at bay, particularly if I was contemplating a pregnancy on Remicade with my recurrent symptoms often requiring Cipro. He wrote me a prescription for a low dose and gave me orders for weekly blood work. I'd see him again in a month's time.

But after a discussion with the pharmacist, I worried about starting the 6-MP. The risks included elevation in liver enzymes, pancreatitis, pancytopenia, lymphoma—scary stuff. After a few weeks of weighing up my options, I decided to give it a go, knowing I was being followed carefully with the weekly blood work.

I started the medication and had no unwanted effects. I was feeling reasonably well, overall. My lab work remained stable with no evidence of elevated liver enzymes, so I continued on a therapeutic dose of 6-MP along with my Remicade. The time between my follow-ups at the GI clinic went from monthly to every twelve weeks.

I stayed healthy through the entire spring. I took a busy work trip to Newfoundland, then took off for Europe the day after getting back; nothing slowed me down. Matt and I travelled to Switzerland and had an amazing holiday, almost like a pre-pregnancy-moon.

With the disease under control, we decided it was time to try to have a baby.

THE IMPACT OF INFLAMMATORY BOWEL DISEASE IN CANADA

*T*he *Impact of Inflammatory Bowel Disease in Canada* (2018) is an important report that was prepared by the scientific community and presented to Crohn's and Colitis Canada. It examines the impact of Crohn's disease and ulcerative colitis across the country. An update of the report published in 2023 found that the general trends reported in the 2018 report, and those forecasting the future, are still holding. The points that follow here—those that particularly resonated with me—have been gleaned directly from the 232-page report.

INCIDENCE RATES, CAUSES, AND RISK FACTORS

Canada has among the highest reported rates of IBD in the world. Approximately 322,600 Canadians—an estimated 1 in 121—live with IBD. An estimated 11,000 people were newly diagnosed with IBD in 2023—one every forty-eight minutes. It

INCIDENCE: The number of new diagnoses of IBD made in a geographic region in a year.

PREVALENCE: The number of people living with IBD in a geographic region at a point in time.

is more than twice as common as multiple sclerosis or HIV and as prevalent as epilepsy and type 1 diabetes.

The *Impact of IBD* report notes that while the incidence of Crohn's disease and ulcerative colitis has stabilized and may be decreasing in western countries, prevalence has continued to rise in Canada. By 2035, it is estimated that 470,000 Canadians—1 in 91—will have IBD.

"Because people are living longer and more people are being diagnosed at a young age, it tends to lead to rising prevalence rates—so, more people [are] living with the disease," says Dr. Jennifer Jones, a team lead of the NSCIBD program at the QEII. "It's a big problem for the healthcare system moving forward."

Nova Scotia has one of the highest reported rates of IBD in the country, which means the province has among the highest incidence of Crohn's and colitis in the world. That includes an estimated nearly 12,000 people in Nova Scotia.

"Why Nova Scotia has the highest rates of IBD, we're not sure, but it's an area certainly of active interest," says Jones. "I suspect it's a combination of our genetics—a lot of Northern European/Celtic-descent individuals—combined with a number of environmental factors. And there may be some that are unique to the province that we haven't completely unearthed or understood yet."

Continents where IBD hadn't largely been diagnosed before 1990—Asia, Africa, and South America, for example—are now experiencing increasing rates of disease.

"We can speculate, based on some of the data and the literature," says Jones. "Historically we've always observed—and this is changing—that in less westernized, less industrial nations, the incidence rates and prevalence rates of IBD were lowest."

The things that come along with industrialization include air pollution, higher levels of processed foods, and more pro-inflammatory diets. When it comes to possible causes and triggers that lead to the onset of Crohn's disease and ulcerative colitis, researchers have discovered that genetics, environmental exposures, and the microbiome are all factors at play. Jones says that in populations that have been well studied so far, genetics only contribute about 10 percent of the risk of developing IBD. "Most likely in individuals who are susceptible there are multiple factors that are contributing to the rising incidence that we're seeing in other countries," she says. "There are studies that show associations between certain dietary components and, for example, items that might be contained in larger amounts in preserved foods—anticaking agents that are added to foods to preserve their shelf life—and those particular food-based exposures actually do have some effect on the mucosal immune system and its response to organisms."

She says more diverse bacteria in our gut is a good thing, but certain types of diets can trigger the growth of a less diverse, more pro-inflammatory group of bacteria in the gut, which could be a risk factor for the development of IBD.

Another component that's been shown repeatedly in the literature, Jones says, is smoking. "We know that cigarette smoking...definitely exacerbates Crohn's disease." Smoking worsens the severity of the disease, blunts response to therapy, and is an independent risk factor in an increased need for surgeries. "We don't see that same effect in ulcerative colitis, but we certainly do see it in Crohn's disease," says Jones. "In that same vein, although it's never been definitively proven in IBD, there certainly are some association studies that look at it for other inflammatory gut conditions."

Jones says researchers also wonder about rising rates of air pollution and poor air quality and whether these factors could be interacting with genetics, diet, and microbiome to raise the risk of developing IBD.

"I think our mucosal-based immune systems are in a fine balance at the best of times because our intestinal tracts are full of bacteria, essentially, and it's up to the mucosal-based immune system to keep things in check," says Jones. "I think it likely doesn't take much—just a few hits probably—to sort of tip that balance and predispose an individual to developing IBD."

Vitamin D deficiency has been hypothesized to increase the risk of developing IBD. This hypothesis stems from the fact that vitamin D is important in regulating the immune system and IBD occurs more commonly in countries in northern latitudes, such as Canada and Scandinavia.

Yet another explanation for the emergence of IBD is the "hygiene hypothesis." This suggests that children growing up in relatively sterile environments—without adequate exposure to microbes—might insufficiently educate their immune systems for handling micro-organisms. They then develop an abnormal immune response that attacks their organs when exposed to harmful micro-organisms. Indirect evidence supporting this hypothesis includes research showing that Crohn's disease and ulcerative colitis are less likely to occur in individuals who live with pets in childhood, are raised on a farm or rural region, have a larger family, or drink unpasteurized milk.

The gut microbiome includes micro-organisms that maintain digestive health. Changes in the microbiome may play a role in IBD. For example, IBD is more likely to develop in people who were exposed to antibiotics within the first year of life and in those who were not breastfed. Antibiotics and breastfeeding strongly influence the diversity of the microbiome in children, laying down the foundation for either the future development of, or protection against, IBD.

Interesting facts from *The Impact of Inflammatory Bowel Disease in Canada* (2018):

- The highest reported incidence of IBD in Canada is in Nova Scotia at 54.6 new cases per 100,000 people per year. The lowest reported incidence is in British Columbia at 18.7 new cases per 100,000 people per year.

- In 2018, 700 out of every 100,000 Canadians had IBD. By 2035, the total number of people living with IBD in Canada is expected to rise to 470,000.

- The age groups most likely to be diagnosed with Crohn's and colitis are adolescents and young adults between the ages of twenty and thirty. Ulcerative colitis is more common in the senior population (over sixty-five), while children are more likely to be diagnosed with Crohn's disease. The general ratio of ulcerative colitis to Crohn's disease in Canada is roughly 50/50 when age is not taken into account.

- The prevalence of IBD in children has risen more than 50 percent in the last twenty years and continues to rise. Increasing incidence of IBD in Canada is primarily driven by pediatric-onset disease, and the number of new cases in this population is quickly rising. The number of annual new diagnoses among those under eighteen years of age, and especially among those under six years old, is the predominant driver of rising incidence.

- Children with Crohn's or colitis have different disease complications, respond differently to treatments, have fewer treatment options available, and are at a greater risk of experiencing side effects of medication as compared to adults.

- Nova Scotia has among the highest rates of pediatric IBD in Canada. Nova Scotia, Ontario, and Quebec have higher rates of pediatric IBD than most countries in the world.
- In 2030, 13,685 children and youth are predicted to be living with IBD in Canada (172 per 100,000 children). This is almost twice the number of children living with IBD in 2018, and almost three times the number living with IBD in 2008.
- Approximately 15% of Canadians with Crohn's or colitis were diagnosed after the age of sixty-five.
- Seniors with IBD are the fastest-growing group of Canadians living with IBD.
- Women are more likely than men to be diagnosed with Crohn's disease in Canada. The risk of being diagnosed with ulcerative colitis is the same for females and males.
- IBD patients cared for by gastroenterologists have better outcomes, including lower risks of surgery and hospitalization. Canadians who live in rural and underserved areas are less likely to be under a gastroenterologist's care, potentially due to care preferences or poorer access, which may result in poorer long-term outcomes.

THE PSYCHOLOGICAL IMPACT OF IBD

D r. Michael Vallis is a registered health psychologist with a focus on chronic diseases: diabetes, obesity, heart disease, and gastrointestinal (GI) disease. Shortly after finishing his graduate work at the University of Western Ontario, he began working with a gastroenterologist at Credit Valley Hospital in Mississauga, ON. When he came to Nova Scotia in 1988 to work in the field of diabetes, he wanted to continue in GI, so he negotiated the opportunity to split his time between the two. He became part of the GI team at the QEII and stayed for thirty years. Now he's mostly teaching and consulting and has developed the Behaviour Change Institute, a training program for lifestyle counselling skills for physicians, nurses, dietitians, and other healthcare providers.

Vallis spent his years on the GI team seeing people with functional gut disorders, liver-related issues, and with his major focus—IBD. Vallis says there are two things about IBD that make it unique in terms of mental health impacts.

"First, you wouldn't wish it on your own worst enemy," he says. "It's a disease with a really huge suffering profile. When someone is symptomatic, the functional impact is really, really intense."

Vallis compares IBD with a disease that is even more intrusive: diabetes, "especially type 1 diabetes, where you might have to make four hundred decisions a day to manage it. But [diabetes] doesn't have the emotional burden attached to it. I mean, it's a pain in the butt. Absolutely. But people adjust." Vallis says once a patient makes it through the adjustment phase of a diabetes diagnosis, they may not be happy about it, but they can take care of it.

"You can actually live incredibly well with diabetes, but IBD…can be brutal, and the extra GI side effects, the fatigue and the malaise, [mean] the suffering profile of the disease is really huge." That is why Vallis thinks it's so important to consider the psychological impact of living with IBD.

"When you see patients presenting with distress…[often] what they're suffering from is their disease. If we took the disease away, they'd be happy as a clam. The rest of the stuff is just called life, and they kind of expect to deal with that. So I think it's actually really important to shine the light on what we call disease-based distress," says Vallis.

Vallis describes himself as a health psychologist. "Most people would know of the typical psychologist who would work with people who have mental health diagnoses," he says. "When you have a mental health diagnosis, it's called psychopathology or pathology of the psyche," he says. "In other words, there's something wrong with you…and a clinical management job is really there to help you. I work with 'normal' people in the 'abnormal' world. Your gut's not supposed to fail you. This isn't your fault; you're not creating this, you're suffering it."

The second point Vallis makes is that he thinks IBD is a very socially isolating disease. "People chat about diabetes and heart disease and cholesterol on the bus, but not [about the fact] that they've had sixteen loose bowel movements that day or are afraid they aren't going to get to the next stop before they soil themselves. [For] people who experience IBD, it's incredibly isolating," he says. "Relationships are taxed because the nature of the illness can take a toll. And depending on how symptomatic [they are], how many episodes, how long is the remission, how many relapses, hospitalization, surgeries—all those things have huge weight [on] the quality of life of individuals living with IBD."

As Dr. Jennifer Jones of the NSCIBD program explains it, IBD affects people's mental health by causing increased levels of distress or anxiety, and researchers now believe that bacteria in the gut may play a part in mental health.

"There is some data from other conditions, like IBS for example, and some early data in IBD, that imbalance of the microbiome may actually release metabolites across the blood–brain barrier and may alter your neurochemistry in the brain," says Jones. "It's still early for IBD, but there are hints that that may be what is going on."

Vallis says this is a fascinating area of research. "We're understanding a lot more about the microbiome and the gut–brain connection, and it seems to be incredibly rich. However, I would put that into a sort of 'developing research' category that hasn't actually translated into clinical practice yet."

Regardless of the underlying cause, Jones says physicians see a high need for mental health care in the IBD population. "It has been probably one of the biggest care gaps that we have struggled with as a multidisciplinary team here in Nova Scotia," says Jones. "Mental health needs in general have historically been limited in terms of access, but that is improving. What we don't really have [are treatments] more tailored to the disease itself."

This is an issue both Jones and Vallis and other members of the NSCIBD team, including nurse practitioners Barbara Currie and Kelly Phalen-Kelly, are working to solve. "The needs of someone living with IBD in relation to mental health interventions…are probably different from the needs of individuals who have other conditions," says Jones, "so we're trying to work on a program that recognizes that and is responsive to those needs. We're calling the program 'IBD Strong.'"

IBD STRONG

Through IBD Strong, the clinic would identify IBD-related distress in a patient through a screening tool. Then they would direct that patient to the appropriate support. Various components of the program will deliver different-intensity interventions to support low, moderate, and severe distress in relation to IBD. Vallis says peer-to-peer support is easiest for patients to access, "so we're really trying to start with that and build from there." The peer support intervention component of the program will see peers being formally trained on evidence-based emotional support. The program will offer informational support, and skills training for self-advocacy and self-management.

The self-management process would guide patients to address some of their issues through an app; they could also access videos on stress and stress management. That kind of support will be enough for many patients, but if a patient needs more, IBD Strong will also address that.

Jones says individuals with the highest need will be able to work one-on-one with a psychologist or psychiatrist. "But we estimate based on the literature that the needs of about 85 percent of our population could likely be met by those first two tiers."

All this is driven by the needs voiced by the patient population, according to Jones. "Also, the design of it, the approach, has been influenced by some qualitative data that we've been able to formally collect from people living with IBD. We didn't just decide this is what we're going to do; we've engaged with patients to make sure that we're on the right track."

Vallis says the primary stumbling block is a lack of resources.

"You can see thirty people a week, and of course you have to see them in follow-up because psychological treatment isn't just a one-off, so you can [only] follow a couple [of] hundred people in a five-year period," he explains. "The numbers are just overwhelming."

The IBD clinic, the nurse navigator, and the nurse practitioners are there to help fill the gap. "So then if a doctor is unavailable," says Vallis, "you can still call Barb or Kelly, and they will run interference [and] find a doctor so that you don't suffer and wait unnecessarily."

UNIQUE CHALLENGES

Nurse practitioner Barbara Currie says the role of mental health in chronic illness is being more and more recognized as a factor that greatly impacts people's daily lives.

"If we consider mental health in general, we know that there's a stigma around mental health, although that is significantly improving in the last many years," says Currie. "People are more and more open, particularly the younger generation, with talking about their mental health. Accessing mental health services has been the greatest challenge. And this is right across the country. ...I think we're making advances, but these are baby steps. They're not going to happen overnight."

Currie says that while IBD patients experience unique anxieties—having accidents, not knowing where bathrooms are, being unable to work, having employers or professors who may not understand the condition—not all IBD-related mental health issues involve anxiety or depression. "What we know is that there is an element of distress related to a change in symptoms, unpredictability of outcomes, the uncertainty of how a treatment is going to work." Currie reiterates that IBD Strong is still in the development stage. In the meantime, there are resources patients can turn to.

"There are existing interventions within the province that are not IBD-specific, but that could very much benefit them," says Jones. "We have community mental health resources and virtual modalities of accessing mental health support."

Vallis says he's confident that somebody living with IBD who reached out to a psychologist on their own would get good care, but it wouldn't be the *best* care, because the therapist wouldn't necessarily understand the disease. "All psychologists know how to do stress management, know how to do psychotherapy, know how to listen, know how to collaborate, know how to empower people," he says. But he remembers being at a meeting where a psychologist was presenting to gastroenterologists and didn't know the difference between a colonoscopy (an examination of the colon via scope) and a colectomy (a surgical procedure to remove all or part of your colon). When it was pointed out that those aren't the same thing, the psychologist said it didn't really matter. Vallis says that was the end of the session.

"The docs just basically said, I am insulted by that and I'm not gonna listen to it," he says. Because as Vallis points out, there's potential for harm if mental health professionals don't know the difference between colitis and Crohn's disease, or they confuse IBS with IBD, or they don't understand what an ostomy means psychologically.

DON'T BE ALONE

Vallis says patients who want help with mental health issues should raise the issue with their doctor.

"Have you ever been in a situation where people make assumptions and then they don't act on something because they assume the other person doesn't want to? It's kind of like that in medicine," he says. "People don't raise issues because they feel like the doctor's in charge, and doctors don't raise these issues because they're not experts on it. ...But doctors are obligated to act on what is presented, and they will. If you raise it...it's their job to come up with a treatment plan."

"The first thing is to talk about it," says Currie. "Talk about it with your family. If you can, talk about it with your primary care provider, your family doctor, or your nurse practitioner. Acknowledge whether there's an underlying anxiety or depression that's being untreated and look for resources that you may forget are there. When you see your primary care provider, ask for a referral to a psychologist for management of your chronic illness. Have that on hand in the event that you decide you're going to look into some private psychological services."

Accessing psychological services privately can be challenging, particularly in terms of cost, if the patient doesn't have coverage within their health plan. But many employers offer employee assistance plans that cover psychological services.

"A lot of people forget about that, or they feel that there's a stigma attached, but they have to remember that it's completely confidential," says Currie. "Find out if you have it and utilize it. If you have coverage through your own plan, utilize private psychological counselling. It's easier to access than community mental health, where you could wait a very long time for assessments."

Currie suggests recognizing limitations and identifying stress triggers, which she acknowledges is easy to say but hard to do for most people, even in the absence of a lifelong chronic illness.

"Make sure you're getting enough sleep, you're getting exercise, you're able to do the things that you enjoy and you're not spending all of your time working," says Currie. "I mean, that goes for everybody. ...I always tell my patients, if they're experiencing a change in their symptoms that's causing them stress, to connect with us at the beginning, not three or four or five weeks into it. Give a call sooner so that we can devise a treatment plan and help reduce symptoms early." Currie says this is what the patient support line for urgent access is for—those times when a patient needs the IBD team quickly.

"Mental health is a very complex combination of a lot of things," says Currie. "It's not just your IBD. It's your work life, your personal life, your family life. It's trying to figure out ways to manage all of that in the background of having a bowel disease. So if some of the other pieces of that puzzle are managed effectively, then the ability to cope with changes in your inflammatory bowel disease is probably going to be better."

Vallis explains that when a person receives a mental health diagnosis, they need one-on-one attentive care. "You need a really intimate relationship to really be trusting and to kind of be poked where you need to be poked," he says. But when mental health is being affected by disease-based distress, he says, "you actually benefit by being in a room with say, eight other people who also have this disease where the psychological treatment isn't so intimate, and you talk about your struggles and you think, 'Oh, thank god other people feel this; this is exactly how I feel.'"

Vallis suggests patients look for support groups like Crohn's and Colitis Canada and the Ostomy Canada Society and seek out Facebook and other groups on social media.

"Don't be alone," he says, reiterating how socially isolating IBD can be.

"I do believe that anything that helps to normalize the experience, [and anything] that could really promote a better understanding and acceptance of those emotional issues and that social component, is really important."

MY STORY:
PREGNANCY—EXPECTING THE
UNEXPECTED (2013–2015)

When we got married, Matt and I knew kids weren't in the picture for us quite yet. We'd married at the fresh age of twenty-five and, sure, we could have continued dating for a while longer, but we believed that since we had already been through so much together, the deal was pretty much sealed. I always said I wanted to have a baby at thirty, and Matt agreed with that timeframe. So we had time. We wanted to enjoy our freedom, our jobs. We worked, celebrated, travelled, and enjoyed our time together as young professional adults. We bought our first house, got our first dog, and we both progressed in our careers. With so many friends leaving the province after graduation, we felt lucky to be working in Halifax.

After we'd been married for a few years, enjoying life as DINKS (double income, no kids) as we liked to say, we decided we were ready to start a family. Rather, we were ready to start thinking about being ready to start a family. We were playing out our lives exactly on schedule—not because we were rigid, meticulous planners, but in part because we had to on account of my health.

One day, because I was involved with Crohn's and Colitis Canada, someone from the marketing team reached out to ask if I had a question for the "Dear Doc" section of their patient publication, *The Journal.* I did.

> I have been married nearly four years and will soon want to think about starting a family. I've had Crohn's disease for fourteen years (I am now twenty-eight years old), have five centimetres left of my colon. I started Remicade two years ago. My treatments have worked their way down to being four weeks apart. Is it safe to conceive and carry a baby while on this much Remicade? How would you recommend I plan for a safe and healthy pregnancy?

The physician's response was this:

> Remicade is an FDA class B drug which means it is generally considered safe in pregnancy although no proper controlled trials have been done (this is very hard to do with any drug in pregnancy). There is an extensive global clinical experience which parallels this class B status and most major IBD centres will continue the drug in pregnancy. However, the drug does cross the placenta and therefore the fetus is exposed to the drug. Therefore, many physicians will attempt to give the last dose at or around 30–32 weeks to minimize exposure in the last trimester and then give another dose immediately postpartum.
>
> …[I recommend that] you have your disease reassessed before attempting to conceive to ensure that you are under good control. If not, alternatives should be explored to ensure you are in remission going into pregnancy. Healthy moms make healthy babies. Ensuring you are in remission, and you are happy taking drugs that have put you into remission are the best bet for a happy, healthy pregnancy.

Healthy moms make healthy babies. This seemed like pretty sound advice to me. We'd already visited the Preconceptual Counselling Clinic through the Perinatal Centre and they'd already agreed to follow me through a pregnancy. My family doctor recommended letting her know three months before we planned to try to conceive. I'd need to stop using birth control at least one full cycle before trying to get pregnant. She wanted me to start taking a prenatal vitamin and top up on folic acid, vitamin B, and vitamin D. If I didn't get pregnant within six months, I was to let her know. Typically, she said, she had women try for a year. But given my health history, she wanted to get ahead of any issues.

In April 2012, she sent me for another quick check-in with the maternal fetal medicine clinic. Dr. Van den Hof let me know he didn't see any reason why we shouldn't have a baby. The blood work they'd ordered showed I had healthy hormone levels, comparable to the range of a teenager, so there was no worry of running out of time at that point. He'd looked at studies involving the medication I took. The available data showed no increase in problems when taking Remicade while pregnant. No harmful effects had been observed in babies up to six months after birth. He put me on more folic acid since, without a colon, it would be harder for me to absorb enough through my diet. Once I was pregnant, it would be deemed a "high-risk pregnancy" and I'd be followed at the Fetal Assessment and Treatment Centre.

Dr. Farina said it seemed like about a third of women felt great IBD-wise, both during and after pregnancy—almost as if pregnancy helped or improved their IBD; a third felt no change; and a third had flare-ups or symptoms, particularly after the baby was born. The best approach was to be in optimal health going into a pregnancy.

It seemed like everything had fallen into place. There was no question: we wanted to have a baby and felt reassured with the green flag from my medical team. We'd done our due diligence. My health was finally decent. It was time.

In the fall of 2012, within two months of trying to conceive and less than a month after my thirtieth birthday, we got a positive pregnancy test result. My family doctor referred us right back to Dr. Van den Hof at the Perinatal Centre at the IWK.

Being followed at the Perinatal Centre was comforting because of all the extra attention, tests, and screenings. It took away the uncertainty any newly pregnant woman might experience. At my first appointment, Dr. Van den Hof noticed an available ultrasound machine and we nipped into an empty room where he did a quick—very early—scan. We could indeed see a healthy sac with a blob of cells. At eight weeks and three days gestation, he could detect a single fetal heartbeat. I got to have an early ultrasound at twelve weeks to confirm everything looked great. I can't imagine having to wait twenty weeks, which is when a typical ultrasound check happens. The perk of having a chronic illness that made my pregnancy "high risk" meant I received extra and thorough care—which brought peace of mind.

When the Christmas holidays arrived, Matt and I invited my family over and had them gather around the Christmas tree for a group photo. As Matt went to take the shot, instead of calling out, "Say cheese!" he shouted, "Say Heather's pregnant!" then caught the chaos that ensued on camera. On New Year's Eve, we told our close friends I couldn't drink any alcohol that year, and they clued in right away with jubilant cheers.

I was seen once a month in the perinatal clinic just a short walk from my workplace. For the twenty-week ultrasound I would be referred upstairs to the high-risk assessment unit where they would take an extra-close look at everything.

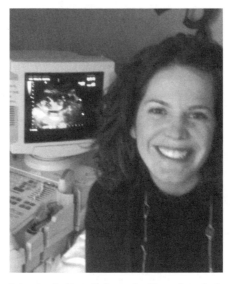

A beaming Heather with her early ultrasound results in
January 2013.

But before I reached that milestone, I wound up back in the
hospital thanks to my Crohn's.

My parents spent their winters in sunny Florida. Matt and
I figured 2013 would be the ideal year to go and visit, while it
was still just the two of us. I was seventeen weeks pregnant. My
Crohn's was under control. Both my GI and family doctors
confirmed there was no risk in flying to Florida at that point.
Whether I was home or away, if something happened with the
baby, there wouldn't be much that could be done to help before
the twenty-week mark.

So we packed our bags. On Friday, March 15, off we went for
an extra-long weekend. With my baby bump finally prominent,
we took photo after photo to capture the memories. We passed
a few lazy days bumming around Sunset Beach. It was perfect.

On the way back home on Tuesday we grabbed tacos with
all the fixings for dinner at a Chipotle restaurant, one of very

few options in the Tampa airport. Matt and I were seated in separate rows on the plane. I had a window seat, next to an elderly man who slept the whole flight. I didn't have the heart to disturb him, so I didn't get up from my seat during the entire flight, despite needing to use the bathroom.

Our flight had been delayed, so it was late when we arrived in Halifax that night; we picked up food at a Wendy's restaurant on the way home. This was the second time I had eaten lettuce that day—something I usually avoided because it was hard for me to digest and could lead to a bowel obstruction. Clearly I wasn't thinking straight.

The next day was stormy and messy outside and I was tired from our late arrival the night before, so I worked from home in the morning. Besides, I noticed I had some pains in my belly. The pain persisted and increased through the day. I knew by the next morning, when I was feeling terrible and hadn't passed anything since Tuesday night, that I needed to get checked out. I managed to get an appointment at the GI clinic with Dr. Farina, who squeezed me in that afternoon. He believed I had either inflammation flaring up or a partial bowel obstruction. He reassured me it had nothing to do with travelling to Florida and that I was lucky this was happening at home and not in the US, where the hospital costs would be astronomical.

My family doctor had told me that if I had any medical emergencies before twenty weeks gestation, pregnancy-related or not, I was to go to the emergency room at the regular adult hospital. After twenty weeks, I'd start reporting to the IWK Health Centre. I was on the borderline, but Dr. Farina made some calls and managed to get me admitted to the IWK so we could get things under control.

He let them know I'd be on my way. We swung home to grab my things—thankfully not yet unpacked from the trip to Florida. I also grabbed a quick shower. I'd played this game before and didn't know when I'd be back in the comfort of my own home.

When I arrived at the IWK triage they determined everything seemed fine, pregnancy-wise. It was indeed likely a Crohn's issue. I was admitted for observation and some treatment—primarily, IV fluids so I didn't wind up any more dehydrated. Even sipping water caused searing pains in my stomach. I wasn't allowed to eat anything. (A pregnant woman, not allowed to eat!) But the pain was so bad I didn't want to eat anyway. When the pain did not subside, I was put on a short-term low dose of prednisone, on the advice that not taking it was a bigger risk than taking it while pregnant, and it would not harm the baby. As always, it did the trick. The inflammation subsided along with the pain, and as soon as I could eat again with no issue, I was sent home. It was Tuesday, March 26. I'd been gone a week and a half longer than the planned "quick long weekend." I weaned off the prednisone right away and had no further issues.

To anyone who asked how the pregnancy was going, my response was always "really great, no problems at all!" But fortunately, I had no other issues, pregnancy-related or otherwise—not even an ounce of morning sickness. My biggest affliction during my pregnancy was an intense craving for any combination of chocolate and peanut butter.

No one on my medical team saw an issue with planning for a vaginal delivery. A scheduled C-section was an option. I decided I wanted to try and see how labour and delivery played out, but if a C-section was necessary, so be it. Matt and I were very much open to going with the flow. We really wanted to defer to the medical team, who we believed knew best. With the pregnancy evolving like any regular pregnancy, my delivery had as much a chance of ending up a C-section as anyone's.

Thanks to the vacation and overtime I'd accumulated, I stopped working three weeks before my due date. I wanted some time to finish preparing for the baby's arrival, and some time to put my feet up. Then, two weeks before my due date, my water broke. Great. I'd just finished devouring a pizza I'd ordered for lunch with my sister and youngest niece.

My labour progressed normally and by that night we were admitted to labour and delivery. My GI doctors had always told me I had a high tolerance for pain and that I tended to downplay my symptoms, but labour contractions brought out a whole new side of me. Once the pains became intense and close together, I turned into a wimp pretty quickly. I tapped out and got an epidural—and to my relief I couldn't feel a thing, which unfortunately then made it difficult to work with the contractions.

After twelve hours of labouring, I started pushing. By early morning, it was time to get the baby out of there. The doctor could see the baby's hair, but the baby would just not budge any further, a shoulder in the way. Then suddenly I was spiking a fever and the baby's heart rate was dropping. There was talk of forceps, which was a no-go for me. I didn't want to unnaturally force anything, with the potential result of tearing that could lead to infection that could become severe because of my medications or other Crohn's complications. It was time for an emergency C-section.

Everything went exactly as it should. Before we knew it, we were in our room upstairs with a brand new, six-pound, thirteen-ounce baby girl with the most outrageous head of hair I'd seen since my own baby photos. Sweet baby Anna had natural highlights on a shock of dark locks standing straight on end. Our little hedgehog, as she affectionately became known.

I may have wimped out on the contractions but recovering from the C-section was a breeze. This was nothing compared to my previous major abdominal surgeries. Plus, I wasn't sick or recovering from a lengthy illness—just soon sleep-deprived and frazzled, like every other new parent.

Dr. Farina's statistic that about a third of women feel great IBD-wise during pregnancy and after, almost as if it helps or improves their disease, proved to be the case for me. My Crohn's was not only vastly improved, it was off my radar. My Remicade dose was delayed by two weeks after delivery while we waited for my C-section incision to heal, but it didn't affect my health. My maternity leave passed by as one of the best years I've ever spent, meeting new mom friends and trying out all the "mommy and me" classes, from mom and baby yoga to Kindermusik and tumblebugs.

Anna was an amazing baby. We had coffee dates with friends, leisurely daily walks, lunches with Matt; she even turned nine months old on the beaches of the Dominican Republic. Life as a new mother was simply the best. I decided not to go back to my old full-time job, opting instead to spend time at home with Anna and building a freelance writing portfolio.

Fast-forward to January 2015. Matt and I decided we were ready to add another person to our family. On Valentine's Day, Matt passed me a bottle of Nova 7, one of my favourite wines. I passed him a positive pregnancy test. We laughed, and I stuck the bottle at the back of the fridge to be enjoyed many months later.

This time around, pregnancy was a little different. I had nausea, though nowhere near the level some of my friends had suffered from. I didn't hesitate to take a daily anti-nauseant medication that made me feel better. Of course, I was also chasing around a two-year-old this time. For a while, my biggest affliction was an intense craving for guacamole, which I hadn't noticed until my niece asked me why I brought it with me everywhere. When I was about three months along, Anna and I, with the baby bump already starting to show, tagged along on Matt's work trip to Los Angeles, extending it into a dream vacation. We toured Hollywood—complete with celebrity sightings—cruised the Pacific Coast Highway, and explored San Francisco. My health remained stable.

Then one morning Matt found me sitting on the kitchen floor at home, slumped against the wall like a rag doll. I literally could not go on. Something wasn't right.

It was June and I had planned to host a summer barbecue at our house with some friends and family. We were celebrating Matt's induction into the Canadian Collegiate Athletic Association's Hall of Fame for his success as a college soccer star; he had won Atlantic player of the year three times, plus national player of the year. It was an accomplishment well worth celebrating. By the day before, we had done a grocery haul at Costco, and I had everything just about ready. But I hadn't been feeling well at all. My bowels weren't functioning properly, and I felt exhausted. The next morning, I tried to press on, getting the house and food ready to host a small crowd, when I had to literally lay down and admit defeat. We cancelled the party so I could rest.

I ended up in the emergency room in the middle of that night because my symptoms felt obstruction-like. I was twenty weeks and six days along, which was around the same point at which I'd had a flare-up during my first pregnancy. I was also achy with chills and a fever. The GI doctor on call suspected an infection. He sent me home and said if things got worse, I'd have a CT scan. I started to feel better as the week went on, but four days later I had to miss the Hall of Fame induction ceremony. Matt, his parents, Anna, and my dad set off for New Brunswick while I stayed behind with my mom for appointments and an ultrasound. It was one of the few times in my life I had to miss something meaningful due to illness (the first being Matt's nineteenth birthday). It left me with pangs of remorse. However, I told myself this one could be chalked up as much to pregnancy as to Crohn's. That was an easier pill to swallow—knowing I had stayed back to ensure the baby's health.

Without intervention, I started to feel better. It was difficult to stay whether it had been a viral gastrointestinal illness or a mild flare-up of Crohn's, but my symptoms improved daily. I proceeded to get my Remicade infusion the next week and continued to feel much better.

Two months later, at twenty-eight weeks pregnant, I fell ill with a sore throat. I felt terrible for a couple of days before finally going to a walk-in clinic for a throat swab—which was faster than getting in to see my family doctor. The doctor at the clinic thought it was a viral infection but tested for strep just in case. I continued to go downhill, lying sick in bed and feeling more and more terrible every hour until my family doctor called the next day to tell me it was indeed strep throat. I needed antibiotics.

I'd been under the weather for a few days and the doctor was concerned that I was getting dehydrated—a big no-no while pregnant. Dehydration can lead to lower levels of amniotic fluid which can influence the baby's development, and it can lead to preterm labour. Being down a colon, I could get dehydrated easily. My doctor told me it was worth heading over to the Early Labour Assessment Unit at the women's hospital to be admitted for IV hydration. They hooked me up to a machine, wrapping a big belt around my waist.

"Do you realize you're having contractions?" the triage nurse asked me.

I hadn't felt anything at all, but I was in preterm labour. It was way too early. I was only twenty-eight weeks pregnant. I was swiftly admitted and put on bedrest. I was given medication to stop the contractions and steroids to strengthen the baby's lungs in case the baby made its arrival early. I was given antibiotics for the strep throat. I subsequently developed a urinary tract infection (UTI) and blood work picked up that my hemoglobin was low. But the name of the game was to stop the contractions and keep the baby inside. Everyone I saw on the medical team said the same thing: "Thirty and flying." If we could get to thirty weeks, there was a much better chance they would be able to take care of everything. The baby would be premature but would have much greater odds of survival.

Once I was admitted to a room, I started to feel the so-called contractions. They were more like a tightening in my abdomen, which is what I called them as I took notes on my phone, recording them every thirty minutes through the evening; they eventually slowed down and finally stopped the next morning.

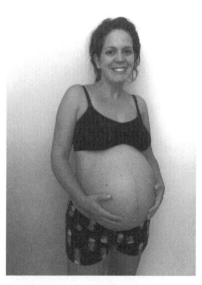

The strep throat cleared up, as did the UTI. After a week, I was sent home with advice to take it easy. I wondered what might have happened if I hadn't gone to labour assessment for what I thought was simple IV hydration. Would I have noticed I was in preterm labour before it was too late? If I had left it too long, could the contractions still have been stopped?

Heather with her big bump for baby number two in September 2015.

Maybe having Crohn's had paid off. It had forced me to pay attention to a seemingly small thing, which turned out to be a much bigger thing.

For this pregnancy, I decided to "treat myself" to a planned C-section, knowing how easy my recovery had been last time. Once again, the decision was mine to make; the doctors were comfortable either way, but I didn't want to go through labour, pushing, *and* a C-section again. In my case, it was also the safest option.

The date was set for the end of October. I was able to choose the date that worked best for us, which seemed comical, as if we'd say, "No, not the Monday; we have dinner reservations." At the next ultrasound, the baby was measuring big, so the date was bumped up by two weeks. I didn't even make it that far.

At my regularly scheduled prenatal appointment at the IWK at thirty-six weeks, I casually mentioned how itchy I was— especially my legs, stomach, and the palms of my hands. I'd been lying awake at night, relentlessly scratching my hands to no relief. The doctor said she was glad I had casually mentioned it because it could possibly be a condition called cholestasis of pregnancy, which is a liver issue. It slows or stops the normal flow of bile from the gallbladder, and it can cause dangerous complications. She couldn't confirm without a blood test but decided to move forward with that diagnosis. She sent me straight for blood work, booked an ultrasound for the next morning, and moved the C-section to the following Monday morning, just five days away.

At the ultrasound the next day everything checked out fine. But the moment we walked back into the house, a strong contraction cramped my abdomen. And then again. I knew I was in labour. We quickly packed some bags, and my parents, who had been watching Anna while we were at our appointment, took her home with them while we headed back to the hospital. The baby was on the way and there was no stopping things.

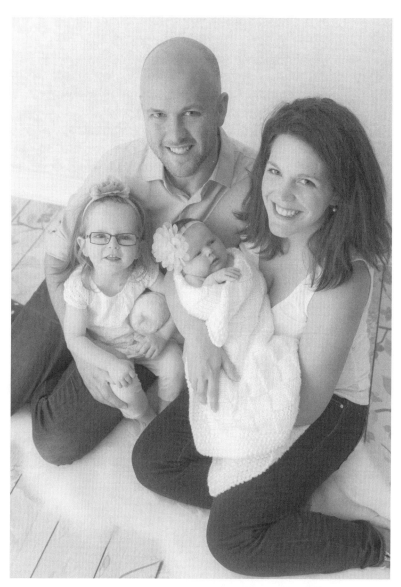

A Fegan family portrait, taken in October 2015, with Matt holding Anna and Heather holding Rosie.

At 7:11 P.M., bouncing baby Rose was born—eight pounds, five and a half ounces—a chubby baby girl with fuzzy brown hair. Our Rosie Posie.

I didn't bounce back from this C-section as smoothly. I had a two-year-old to contend with and it wasn't long before I thought that this time I might be in the one-third of women whose Crohn's flares up after having a baby.

I didn't feel great throughout the fall, with minor symptoms here and there—mostly digestive issues and obstruction-like symptoms. By January, with a two-year-old toddler and a three-month-old baby at home, and in the midst of trying to sell our house, I had a full-blown flare-up.

I landed back in the hospital once again.

CROHN'S IN THE FAMILY

While Crohn's disease is known to have a genetic link, the genetic elements that cause Crohn's to develop in some people are not fully understood. Observation suggests that environmental factors are likely to be of much greater importance than genetics in driving the emergence of IBD.

My father was an aircraft electronics technician and a logistics officer in the Royal Canadian Air Force. Military transfers had our family constantly moving across Canada. My brother, Donnie, was born in Belleville, ON, in 1967; my sister Debbie was born there in 1969. My sister Denise was born in Germany, where my family was stationed, in 1975—long before I arrived. I was born in Cold Lake, AB, in 1982, moving across the country (via Winnipeg) and landing in Nova Scotia by the time I was five.

Three out of four of us have been diagnosed with Crohn's disease, but it's difficult to discern why. Clearly something has predisposed some of us. Yet all my siblings and I have been exposed to the same environmental factors; we share genes and are descended from the same Northern European Celtic lineage.

But as with many things around Crohn's—the true cause remains a mystery.

DONNIE

After me, my brother has the next most severe Crohn's disease in the family.

Over the past forty-five years, Donnie has spent time living in Belleville; Trenton, ON; Baden, Germany; Victoria, BC;

Kingston, ON; back to Trenton; Cold Lake, AB; Winnipeg, MB; then back to Victoria and Kingston for Royal Military College; and on to Ottawa, Calgary, Halifax, and then back to Ottawa in 2012, where he currently resides. Having also joined the military, various deployments have taken him to the United States, Croatia, the Middle East, and Haiti. Not exactly a smooth, stable, or stress-free lifestyle. In terms of international locations, deployments with the military could mean environmental conditions and a lack of dietary options that may have contributed to health problems. When he was deployed, he would have had to eat the food they had on offer so it would have been almost impossible for him to regulate his symptoms by eating different foods.

Donnie always had a sensitive stomach as a kid, with his stomach aches often attributed to food just not agreeing with him.

"Mom will confirm that teachers told her I always said I had a tummy ache for some reason," he says. "It never slowed me down; I was an extremely active kid, especially with sports."

His main trouble started as an adult. In 1991, at the age of twenty-four, he had a night of severe stomach pain and vomiting that landed him in the hospital overnight. "Apparently the doctors initially thought I was going through some kind of withdrawal from drugs. I was put on IV and released the next day. No diagnostics were conducted."

This became an annual event for Donnie, where at least one night a year he would have severe stomach pain and vomiting. It continues to this day on an annual basis.

Sometime in 1997 he saw military doctors to try and find out why this was happening. He had a colonoscopy that revealed nothing. He considered asking for a lactose intolerance test, but milk didn't always bother him, so he didn't.

In the past, Donnie had been a very casual cigar smoker, stopping altogether ten years ago. "I smoked a little in Croatia with a buddy because it was pervasive and helped us fit in when near the locals," he says. "It was wartime all around and seemed like a thing to do based on all the cool people in war movies we'd seen."

He admits that, growing up, he ate too much fast food. "I ate at McDonald's for lunch every day during the last two years of high school." As an adult, his diet consisted of a lot of red meat and processed food ("the bachelor diet," as he calls it), with wine and beer on the weekends.

"I kept having stomach issues, and when I deployed to Haiti in 2010, I was sent with six months' worth of prescribed Zantac and another prescription of mefloquine for malaria," he says, noting he's now part of a class action lawsuit over the military's use of mefloquine without full disclosure of possible serious side effects. Zantac use has also been linked to long-term issues, and he used it multiple times per day throughout the deployment.

By the spring of 2015 Donnie was having trouble with his bowels and feeling extremely fatigued. This had an impact on his fitness regime; he had been very active, working out or playing sports most days of the week. Now he was running out of breath after simply walking for extended periods. He would sometimes black out if he stood up quickly. In June 2015 he ran a half marathon—very slowly and walking much of the way, to his great dismay.

"On July 15, 2015, I went to the military hospital to get checked out, assuming it was a blood pressure issue," he says. "I was extremely tired all the time. They did a blood test in the afternoon and I went back to work to get ready to go home. I got a call from a doctor as I was heading to the bus and he asked if I was bleeding. Confused, I said that I didn't think so. He said that my hemoglobin was dangerously low and I needed to get to a hospital for emergency blood transfusions as soon as possible."

He had the transfusions at a civilian hospital that night and was sent home the next day with a colonoscopy and upper endoscopy scheduled for two days later. When the scopes revealed nothing, he went through various other tests and scans over almost three months. A CT scan ultimately showed what could be signs of Crohn's. "The GI doctor then decided to use a children's scope and found an ulcer in my ileum—and formally diagnosed me with Crohn's."

The diagnosis came as no surprise to his family—we had all diagnosed him with Crohn's years before that, based on family experience.

Donnie's initial treatment in October 2015 started with Pentasa (one of the 5-ASA medications), along with daily doses of iron and B-12. The vitamin doses continue to this day. Taking antacids help with periodic acid reflux and indigestion.

Eventually, the Pentasa stopped helping. Yearly scopes showed that the ulcer was still there. His gastroenterologist put him on Imuran and a short course of prednisone. By 2019 he was needing repeated balloon dilations to open strictures (narrowing of the bowel) during his annual scopes, and the ulcer remained. That fall he made the jump to biologics. His doctor put him on Humira on a biweekly basis, and it seemed to help.

Interestingly, that year he spent over five months (from October to March) in Portugal eating a Mediterranean diet and says he felt better than he had in years. When he returned to Canada in 2020, he says his issues—periodic pain, days of frequent bowel movements—returned.

"In the spring of 2022 I had my first scope in over three years and another stricture had to be repaired. By June I was having severe bloating and pain on a regular basis." His doctor doubled his Humira dosage. A November colonoscopy revealed yet another stricture. "The doctor tattooed the spot, presumably to show where I may need surgery if the stricture keeps reoccurring."

Since his Crohn's diagnosis, Donnie's diet has consisted of more home-cooked and fewer fast-food meals, no beer, and less wine. "I drink oat lattes and take Lactaid now before consuming dairy products," he says. "I can't say enough good things about a Mediterranean diet, thanks to my stint in Portugal."

Donnie says stress is a big trigger for his Crohn's symptoms. "My last military job as a colonel from 2015 to 2019 was very stressful, so it created more pain and suffering than I might otherwise have had," he says.

Donnie is now retired from the military; his medical status indicated he was no longer deployable, and a medical early release was possible. He is now working as a civilian for the Department of National Defence as manager of pension policy. "I work from home and have a team of six," he says. "It's a much slower pace and less stressful—most of the time."

Donnie says the repaired stricture and informal prescription of Lactaid seemed to make things much better. Nevertheless, a worsening of symptoms soon prompted his doctor to switch his prescription to a bimonthly infusion of a different biologic drug called Stelara (ustekinumab). He still has days of fatigue and stomach issues that he treats with antacids.

"I am trying to get back in shape with hockey, snowshoeing, and cross-country skiing, as my fitness regime basically stopped in June 2022," he says. "Age and years of sports and military injuries don't help."

Donnie intends to travel as long as his health will allow. He plans to get back to the Mediterranean lifestyle and the diet that supports his health so well—thanks to a newly purchased condo in the Algarve region of Portugal.

DENISE

My sister Denise has mild to moderate Crohn's that she's been able to keep in remission.

After being born in Lahr, Germany, she moved across Canada with the family to various locations before moving back to Halifax, where she currently resides.

Growing up, she led a relatively healthy lifestyle, with periods of regular exercise. She was a smoker from the age of nineteen until she was twenty-four.

Denise began having IBS symptoms and became lactose intolerant at around nineteen, and within four or five years her symptoms got worse, becoming more frequent after her first and second pregnancies.

She had her first scope at age thirty, which showed lesions and ulcers as well as strictures and red, irritated inflammation at the terminal ileum that wouldn't allow the scope to pass. She was diagnosed then with Crohn's disease.

Denise started out trying various anti-inflammatory medications (5-ASAs) and a corticosteroid called Entocort (budesonide). The Entocort was very helpful to settle flares, but the 5-ASA medications were not working. She started the immunosuppressive drug Imuran that same year and has been on it ever since, with a few small adjustments to the dose along the way. She had to go on steroids a few times over the first few years to help get things under control.

Denise had a restricted diet for years, with no fruit or vegetable skins and no seeds or insoluble fibre. She's tried various diets, the most successful involving cutting back sugar and carbohydrates after blood work detected elevated sugar levels and inflammation markers; the diet resulted not only in weight loss, but also in helping to lower her inflammation levels.

Denise has been on Imuran for seventeen years now and has been in full remission for the last few. She recently met with her gastroenterologist and discussed coming off the drug sometime in the next few years because the Imuran is suppressing her immunity to everything else. If things continue to go well, she'll have a scope in a year or two, then decide.

DEBBIE

Unlike the rest of us, my oldest sister, Debbie, does not have Crohn's disease—but that doesn't mean she is free of digestive and autoimmune issues.

Debbie avoided milk and dairy products when she was younger because they gave her terrible stomach pains. She could handle a little pizza and ice cream, but never at the same time. She found chocolate milk was easier to digest, even putting it on her cereal—much to our mother's chagrin. Today she religiously takes a lactase enzyme when she consumes dairy products but that's as far as her gastrointestinal issues have gone.

Debbie has never smoked and has lived a fairly active lifestyle. About ten years ago, she became vegetarian after a one-month challenge from her teenaged son rolled into a full-on lifestyle change.

Interestingly, Debbie has suffered from a disease called keratoconus (KC), an eye disease that affects the structure of the cornea, characterized by the thinning of the cornea and irregularities of the cornea's surface, resulting in loss of vision.

As with IBD, the cause is unknown, but KC is believed to occur due to a combination of genetic and environmental factors. One study shows some strong associations between KC and autoimmune diseases which may point to the role of the immune system.

Debbie was fitted for special custom contact lenses, but her left eye continued to thin and scar and eventually a cornea transplant was required. "The outcome was amazing; up close I can see clearly without a lens, but I still require [contact] lenses. My left cornea is now over eighty years old."

MY STORY: PARENTHOOD, PAIN, AND PANIC ATTACKS (2016–2019)

In January 2016 Matt and I decided to get our house ready to put on the market ahead of the spring real estate season. There wasn't much inventory for sale, and our realtor said people looking for houses in the winter are often hungrier because they *have* to make a move. We lived in a property in a historic neighbourhood built out of the ashes of the Halifax Explosion, and we wanted more space—a bedroom of her own for the baby (Anna's being way too small to share), and space to set up a home office for my freelance work.

Our realtor helped us come up with a great plan. We'd get the house staged and ready for viewings, and rather than trying to keep the place looking meticulous (and empty at a moment's notice for viewings) we'd stay at my parents' place while they spent the bulk of the winter in Florida.

A home stager suggested putting most of our belongings into storage. We were hard at work decluttering as much as we could and packing up anything we didn't really need for the time being. We marked things with sticky notes—keep, get rid of, storage. We planned to swap out some of the furniture and artwork and really glam the space up. A fresh coat of paint, the whole works.

I had started feeling unwell, with crampy pains in my gut all the time. I was exhausted and my digestive system wasn't working properly; it often seemed like nothing was passing through. I pressed on, but not without calling the GI clinic, where I managed to get an urgent appointment with a nurse practitioner.

At the appointment I told her everything that was going on. She took notes for my file, which Dr. Farina would see later. We discussed the issue of dehydration, and she suggested I increase my fluid intake. She agreed it seemed like it could be the rumblings of a partial bowel obstruction, and said I should watch my diet carefully, be sure to hydrate, and add lots of sodium to help with hydration. At this stage I was breastfeeding, so I didn't want to introduce any medications, knowing full well the suggestion would be a round of prednisone. I never wanted to be on that drug again, let alone while I was breastfeeding. We also discussed reassessing my Crohn's. She'd talk to Dr. Farina about scheduling an MRI of my pelvis; in the meantime she ordered blood work and sent me on my way. I did not feel super confident about the plan of action leaving that appointment, but I also desperately wanted to get on with things. What else could we do? I stopped at the drugstore to fill my pseudo-prescription of cans of sodium-rich chicken noodle soup.

Two weeks later, still struggling with my health, I bundled myself and the kids up on a snowy Friday afternoon and headed out to my mom-and-baby yoga class. It was an ideal situation. My parents, not yet in Florida, lived near the yoga studio and I was able to drop Anna at their place on the way. I could then spend some focussed quality time with Rosie, something I rarely had the chance to do.

I wasn't feeling well that afternoon, but I thought the stretching and de-stressing might help. The roads weren't great, but we made the trek. I pulled up to the yoga studio, heaved the heavy bucket seat out of the back of the car, and went to head inside with a miraculous few minutes to spare before the class started.

The front entrance was locked. A handwritten note on the door apologized for any inconvenience and said the class had been cancelled. There was no one there. I was left fuming out in the cold. Surely this kind of cancellation warranted a phone call! Anyone with young kids knows how hard it is to get out the door. To do it while feeling unwell and in poor weather conditions was a tremendous undertaking. It felt like a real kick in the (already sore) gut.

Determined not to allow my time to be wasted, I decided to tackle a task on our to-do list instead. I went to a self-storage place to figure out the best solution for storing the stuff from our house. We could start moving things over that weekend.

I soon found myself being escorted down a seemingly endless hall, passing door after door of storage units under glaring fluorescent lights, carrying an eight-pound car seat with a fifteen-pound baby in it. The employee was touring me through the company's wide range of storage options: various sizes, indoor access, outdoor access, heated options, the whole shebang. Meanwhile, I was having tight cramps and stabbing pains, gritting my teeth and bearing it. I was dehydrated, I was weak, and I was wondering what on earth I was doing there roaming around.

But getting things done was what I was doing. I wrote down all the information I apparently needed there and then. While essentially weightlifting. In the middle of a Crohn's flare. In the middle of a snowstorm.

Anyone who didn't have Crohn's disease would not have been out doing this in such a state. They'd have been home in bed—or maybe in the emergency department waiting to be checked out. But I didn't have time to stay in bed every time I didn't feel well. When you feel unwell when you have Crohn's disease, you have a pretty good idea of what's going on—your Crohn's is going on. I didn't need to go to the emergency room to be told that. I figured I'd be all right in a few days. I had to push through when I could.

Armed with all the information I needed I made my way to pick up Anna and headed home. Friday was pizza night. We made delicious homemade pizza and I enjoyed a cold cranberry ginger ale. I probably shouldn't have been drinking something bubbly, but I was craving it. We watched *Annie*, the original movie, and Anna was mesmerized by what would soon become an obsession.

That night was excruciating. I woke up over and over with pain. We knew in the morning I had to get checked out. My sister came to pick me up and we headed to the Cobequid Health Centre, a small hospital in a suburb of the city, with the hope that I could be seen sooner there than I might be at the QEII. I wanted to get home to nurse the baby as soon as I could. I figured they could hydrate me with IV fluids, prescribe an anti-inflammatory, things would settle down, and I'd be out of there. That's always the hope—not always the outcome. We left Matt behind with a container of formula that had arrived unbidden in the mail and had been stashed in the back of the cupboard—just in case.

At the emergency room, they took me in right away—a "perk" of having blood pressure that gets dangerously low when I'm dehydrated. While I was waiting, things got worse. The pain intensified and my belly bloated. An abdominal X-ray showed air-filled loops of bowel; the doctors could not rule out an obstruction.

They decided to do a CT scan, but first I had to drink a large cup of a disgusting liquid. I threw it straight back up, apologising profusely to the nurse. The CT scan showed significant bowel-wall thickening and active inflammation causing a partial small-bowel obstruction. I needed a nasogastric (NG) tube immediately, which was inserted through my nose and directly into my stomach to suction out air to decompress my bowel. I would need additional treatment and I would not be going home. The only place I was going was to the hospital in the city, where I was transported by ambulance.

I was admitted to a room shared with an elderly man I never actually saw—we both kept our curtains closed but were mere feet apart in the small hospital room. I was taken off all food and drink. My chart read "nothing by mouth" or NPO, which is the medical shorthand from the Latin *nil per os*. (If I'd thought doctors telling a pregnant woman she was on bowel rest and could not eat—no food whatsoever—had been wild, I'd clearly never imagined them telling a breastfeeding post-partum mother she's on bowel rest and could have no food. Yikes. Doctors really are brave.) I had an IV line inserted for fluids and to receive medication to reduce the inflammation. Solu-Medrol is a corticosteroid similar to prednisone that can be given at higher doses as an infusion for treatment of severe inflammation. Steroids were the only thing that always worked, without fail, but they were not an ideal solution for someone who was breastfeeding.

The doctors thought it would be okay if I continued nursing Rosie. This meant I'd need to pump around the clock to prepare enough milk for her while we were apart. I'd been pumping here and there over the past couple of months, storing up milk for the occasional bottle. There was no way I was going to be able to produce enough to supply all her feedings—not at the best of times and certainly not in my current state. Plus, what if the milk ran out while I wasn't there, a real-life nightmare in the middle of the night? Matt and I had already made an impromptu decision to start her on formula when I'd left for the emergency room. She'd need to continue on a bottle; thankfully, she would take it. But I could pump to at least supplement her feedings and keep my supply up for when I was feeling better.

I provided Matt a list with all the things I needed for my stay—this time around including a breast pump, extra bottles, storage containers, and a bottle sterilizer. That was a first for my hospital bag.

My sister loaned me a small Coca-Cola–branded mini fridge for my hospital room so I could store milk. It was quite a sight—like I was trying to bling up my dorm room. I set a timer: every three hours, day and night, while I wasn't allowed to eat or drink anything, I pumped milk. It was thin, watery milk with a greenish tinge. I knew there was no way I would be feeding it to my baby, but I still stored it in the mini fridge. I kept pumping to keep my supply up. Doctors would come in on their rounds and find me pumping. Nurses would come to adjust the IV pump in the middle of the night and I'd be pumping away.

One day a nurse offered to move me across the hall to a big private room—a double room with only one bed, where I'd have more space to visit with the girls and more privacy to pump. A private room in the hospital is *everything*. It's a luxury (relatively speaking, of course), and it makes a world of difference, but it is not often an option. After a couple of quiet nights on my own, a nurse reluctantly told me I'd need to move back across the hall. She felt bad about moving me again but needed the room for an end-of-life patient.

Of course I didn't mind being sent back to my old room— and old roommate. It was one of those fresh-perspective moments. Being in the hospital, unable to eat, pumping around the clock, away from the girls—one of them a three-month-old baby—really sucked. But I'd get better and I'd be home soon. The patient across the hall would not be leaving the hospital. Their family would be leaving without them, forever.

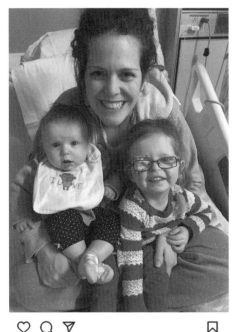

♡ ◯ ✈   🔖

29 likes

theheatherchronicles Going on day five in the hospital tomorrow (I'm ok, Crohn's just decided it was time to become reacquainted, in a big way). These two gems are the best medicine in the world. I mean look at my face. Does that look like the face of someone who's been terribly ill and hasn't had a single bite of food since Friday? Ok maybe, but it doesn't matter where I am in the whole wide world with them on my lap, even just for an hour. Counting down the seconds until I'm home sweet home with them!! (And Matt of course, who's been bouncing between work, home, and hospital and I don't quite understand how he's still on his feet!) ♥♥♥

Heather's February 2, 2016, @theheatherchronicles Instagram post

---

But we were still in the midst of preparing to list the house. My family—big, boisterous, and loud but supremely organized, by way of a military upbringing and numerous moves across the country over the years—sprang into action and decisions were made. Matt and the girls would make an early move to my parents' place so Matt could have support with the girls and childcare at the ready so he'd be able to get to the hospital to see me. We'd stick to our schedule of moving things over to storage that weekend but make the move to my parents at the same time, a week earlier than planned.

On Sunday, the day after I was admitted to hospital, and thanks to the work already done on our part to prepare, my siblings and parents helped move all the items to the thoughtfully selected storage unit I'd booked two days earlier mid-bowel obstruction. Anything with a "storage" sticky note was whisked away. Resting in bed at the hospital, I could only imagine the precision operation that was under way.

"This is weird, moving things out of the house without Heather here," Matt said at one point, as my sister later confided to me. "It's like she's dead." I'm sure he filed that notion away under morbid thoughts he'd never thought he'd have.

After twenty-four hours, a nurse removed the NG tube. I was responding well to the IV Solu-Medrol and after four days transitioned to oral prednisone pills. I was gradually introduced back to eating, starting with clear fluids and working my way up to a soft diet. As soon as I could tolerate food, I'd be on my way home. After six days in hospital, I was to be discharged. It was early Friday morning. Bottle by bottle, I dumped all the pumped milk into the bathroom sink, watching all my hard work swirl away down the drain. I gathered my things and Matt came to pick me up. We headed home, only this time to my parents' place—my childhood home. We got there just in time for breakfast.

I rented a medical-grade breast pump and managed to keep up my milk supply. As soon as I started weaning off the prednisone, I went back to nursing the baby. Prednisone is a difficult drug—the side effects are terrible. But it's also a miracle drug. It helps me feel significantly better right away, every time. I had more energy and felt more like myself. With the help of my mom we finished packing up the rest of the odds and ends at the house.

The painters started on schedule and the next week my sister helped me stage our home with new accessories, furniture, and borrowed artwork. By the time we were done it looked so good I questioned why we were even moving anymore. Then I remembered a good percentage of our belongings were spread between a storage unit and a second home and the only space for our three-month-old was a bassinet beside our bed.

Life carried on. Shortly after I was discharged from the hospital, Matt, the kids, and I took a winter getaway with a group of friends to a cabin just outside the city. (They were so kind, giving us the biggest room so we'd be the most comfortable after everything we'd just been through.) Our house went on the market. My parents left on their winter travels. We settled into life in suburbia. And for the second time in my life, my hospital stay earned me a trip to Florida. Matt, feeling bad for me after my whole hospital ordeal, booked us flights to visit with my parents for a long weekend, much as we had when expecting Anna. Only this time, the obstruction was over before we took the trip.

That March I saw Dr. Farina for a follow-up. I also had the MRI that had been suggested back in January to reassess the disease activity. The scans showed the typical bowel thickening that always seemed to be there, and inflammation in the same old spot. I was tapering off the prednisone, lowering the dose week by week. To avoid another flare-up, he increased my dose of Remicade and kept the frequency at every four weeks.

That spring we bought a new house, sold our old house, and moved—all within a week. Things were really turning around.

One week after moving in, we left for an amazing two-week holiday to Italy, where Matt's sister got married, and thankfully my body behaved. Everything was smooth sailing until a couple of months later when a gastro bug hit our home, with significant consequences.

In hindsight, it's no surprise things unfolded the way they did. I had worn myself out. After returning from the holiday in Italy we'd started a significant renovation on our new place. It might have been a bit ambitious to rip up the main floor of the house we'd just moved into while living there with a three-year-old and a nine-month-old. Walls were torn down, doorways were widened, and we had a bathroom installed on the main floor. We set up a makeshift kitchen in the basement and lived there through the renovation.

During the first week of July Matt came down with a mild stomach bug. Over the weekend, we threw Anna a big third birthday party, hosted at my in-laws' place for lack of space at our own. We picked up pizza on the way home and ate it in the basement. It was that Saturday night that I started feeling an upset stomach.

Our attempt to live in a construction zone with two small children was valiant. We finally abandoned ship and decided to go stay with my parents (again!) while our home was in the thick of construction. I could only corral the kids away from the hub of our home for so long before exhaustion kicked in. Over the next few days, as we settled in at my parents, it felt like I had a long, overdrawn gastro bug, albeit a fairly mild one.

We were set to leave on Thursday, July 14 (our wedding anniversary, no less) on a road trip to Poland Spring Resort in Maine to celebrate my parents' fiftieth wedding anniversary with my whole family. We had T-shirts reading "McLeod Family: Established 1966" made for everyone. I was working on a surprise newsletter with stories and greetings from people who had been in my parents' lives over the years. With two days to go, I laid on the bed in the spare bedroom, feeling completely nauseous and half asleep, designing the document on my laptop. I woke up on July 13, Anna's birthday, feeling very dehydrated. I hadn't been eating or drinking enough; I was depleted from breastfeeding Rosie, who was nine months old. It took everything I could muster to make it to the living room, where we gave Anna her present—a Journey Girl doll that looked just like her. The resemblance was almost uncanny—right down to the glasses, blue eyes, straight brown hair, and facial features. The gift of a "twinsie" was a hit. ("Dana," as she was called, was part of our family for years—one of Anna's favourite toys, but to me, a continuous reminder of that crappy day.)

With the plan to leave for the US the next morning, and at the urging of my mother, we decided I should pay a visit to the emergency room for hydration. Without a colon to absorb water into my system, I always had a hard time catching up after being sick. I didn't want to go downhill while I was out of the country, and I wasn't improving at all after four days of being unwell. I felt terribly guilty to leave Anna on her birthday, but I figured we'd be back in a few hours. Besides, she was in great hands with her grandparents. Matt took me to the Cobequid Health Centre, where I'd first headed when I was sick six months earlier, once again hoping to be in and out quickly. We got there at 10:50 A.M., explaining I had the same gastro-like illness my husband had the week before.

Coincidentally, the cake mix I'd used to make Anna's cake for her party a few days earlier had been recalled due to an *E. Coli* outbreak, but none of our guests had fallen ill so it seemed unlikely to be the culprit. I mentioned this nonetheless. After receiving my obligatory IV fluids and a round of blood work, my glucose levels came back low and my electrolytes off, further proof of my dehydration. I was medicated for nausea. My blood pressure remained low, so I was given more fluids.

More blood work to check on the electrolytes, then a third round of fluids. With my nausea improved and only intermittent pains in my stomach, I was assessed for discharge. The IV line was removed and I was free to leave the emergency room at 4:35 P.M., mission seemingly accomplished. The visit had taken five and a half hours, which was longer than I'd anticipated. I was anxious to get home and reunite with the birthday girl, and to pack everything up for our departure in the morning.

As I gathered my things and changed from the all-too-familiar johnny shirt into my own clothes, a sudden severe pain stabbed at my abdomen.

"Something's wrong," I suddenly groaned. "My stomach!" I was panting.

"Can we get a hand here?" Matt called out, flagging a nurse who called back the doctor who ordered a set of X-rays. Within twenty minutes I was in the X-ray department ready for an abdominal series. The pictures showed "dilated loops of small bowel containing air-fluid levels suspicious for distal obstruction." It looked like I had a partial bowel obstruction. My blood pressure was dropping again, so the IV line was reinserted and fluids started back up. A CT scan was ordered.

A nurse gave me a powerful painkiller—Dilaudid (hydromorphone)—which I knew would knock me out.

"You should go have dinner with the birthday girl," I insisted to Matt as the drowsiness kicked in. My mom came in to keep an eye on me. I was devastated about missing the party as Matt headed off to take the girls to dinner and I drifted in and out of sleep on my stretcher.

It wasn't until 6:35 P.M. that I had the CT scan. The findings were "consistent with obstruction likely related to a combination of active inflammation and chronic stricturing given the long-standing disease in this location."

By 7:30 P.M. I need more pain medication and the doctor decided he wanted to insert an NG tube through my nose to suction the air out of my stomach to try and decompress my bowel. It became obvious I wasn't going home—or to the Poland Springs Resort—and an ambulance was ordered to transport me to the QEII for admission.

As they'd planned, the other fourteen members of my family—minus Matt and the kids—set off for the big anniversary trip. I'd rarely let being sick stop me from doing anything, but I didn't have the choice to push through this time. My Crohn's disease meant I had to miss out on the big event. The NG tube in my nose literally had me tethered to the wall. There was nothing to do but surrender.

I had to be treated with bowel rest and prednisone. After a consultation with both the GI team and general surgery, I underwent a procedure under general anesthetic called ileorectal anastomosis dilation, using air to widen the bowel. It was performed by a surgeon I hadn't met before—but one I would meet again.

I'm typically a pretty patient patient but on this admission I begged to have the NG tube removed. "I don't want you to bring the girls to visit until this thing is out," I told Matt. It wasn't a nice experience, and I didn't want Anna to be frightened by the shocking site of it. Thankfully it was removed after a few days.

I was also anxious to be discharged.

"When can I go home?" I asked the doctor following my care.

"Once you can tolerate food, you can be discharged," he promised.

The first meal sent to my bedside was a thick steak smothered in a foul-looking gravy. So much for a soft diet. What a joke. I convinced the doctor I could feed myself a much more appropriate diet at home and he couldn't argue with that. With a bit of hesitation from him (he wanted one more day) and a promise that I knew what I was doing by now, he let me go. It was, after all, not my first rodeo. With my meds switched from IV to oral tablets, I was discharged on July 18 after six days in hospital, once again returning to my parents' place to recuperate until the bulk of our home reno was complete.

There were no complications in the days that followed, and I was feeling well overall. The prednisone was doing the trick.

A week later, at a follow-up appointment with my gastroenterologist, I was given the go-ahead to start tapering off, reducing the dose week by week until I got off it all together.

By August we were back to living in our own house but still navigating the last bits and pieces of the renovation. One sunny morning, the girls and I were waiting for my sister-in-law and nephew to come over. We were going to go for a walk on the nearby trail. One minute I was sweeping the kitchen floor (we now had cabinets, but no countertops) and the next instant I did not feel well at all. It hit me like a wave. Pain washed over my gut and my back, nausea rippling through me.

Quickly, I stuck Anna in front of the TV and ran with Rosie to her nursery, calling Matt at work.

"You need to come home and help me. Something's wrong—my stomach," I moaned into the phone.

"I'm on my way," he replied, no questions asked.

I then called my sister—whose workplace is closest to our house—and asked her to come quickly to watch the kids. Writhing in pain in the rocking chair, I quickly nursed Rosie to placate her and stuck her in the crib, then dashed out of her room to vomit. Something was *very* wrong.

It wasn't long before Matt and I were on the way to the emergency room, positive it was yet another bowel obstruction. I was quickly triaged and sent to the waiting room, where I couldn't even sit down. I paced the floor, and in a move completely out of character for me, charged back to the desk, hollering for help. I was whisked off to a bed and given fentanyl, the powerful opioid, which offered near-instant relief, along with Gravol for the nausea. By the time the doctor came to see me almost two hours later, he already had an answer as to what was going on.

"I was able to review your CT scan from last month," he said. "There is a very small spot far to the right side, a renal calcification." A kidney stone. He sent me off for X-rays, which showed there were now two rounded calcifications in my pelvis. The stones were on their way out, which explained everything. The doctor told me they would pass on their own and sent me on my way with two more rounds of painkillers—Dilaudid this time—to see the kidney stones through. I spent the rest of the day drugged up on the couch watching the Summer Olympics, grateful to have a bit of rest. The next day it was back to my regularly scheduled programming, a bowel obstruction avoided.

Later that summer I had a follow-up appointment with the surgeon who had overseen my procedure during the last hospital admission. The report said:

> Remicade and 6-MP made her Crohn's quiescent for the most part over these years. Unfortunately, increasingly over the last 12–24 months she has had episodes of partial small bowel obstructions. Most recently, she presented in the context of a gastrointestinal infection, or so she thought, to Cobequid, where there was quite marked dilation of the small bowel with narrowing...she was transferred and examined and it was felt that she did in fact have a stricturing that was the etiology of the small bowel obstruction.

The report went on to say I needed further examination under anesthesia, and I was to be booked for an endoscopy and flexible sigmoidoscope to assess the disease and everything that was going on. The report also mentioned the potential fate I'd been avoiding:

> We did discuss with her today that at the end of the line, her only option if this becomes increasingly symptomatic, would be complete proctectomy and end ileostomy. ... [But] at this time, with good function, there is no need to rush into that and we will start with an examination and characterization of this stricture and her anatomy."

This surgeon had a much more reasonable attitude. I felt like I'd dodged yet another bullet.

With the prednisone having worked its magic again, the next months passed by with only one minor blip—another trip to the emergency room in November due to dehydration after a bout of gastroenteritis complete with fever, aches, sore throat, and vomiting. No abdominal pain or obstruction, just cramps and nausea, so a dose of Zofran (ondansetron)—a strong anti-nauseant that's effective for treating gastroenteritis—and IV fluids left me feeling better and on my way without a hospital admission.

I received no word regarding appointments for the follow-up exams and scopes that had been ordered by the doctor that summer. Wait-lists in the healthcare system were long, but that didn't matter much to me because I was back in remission and feeling well.

Then along came March 2017. Anna came down with a stomach bug, which I tried my best to avoid. I was not the front-line parent when it came to contagious illnesses like that, for good reason. I tried to avoid germs like the plague itself, for fear of exacerbating my Crohn's or ending up with severe dehydration. Her illness was short-lived, as these things tend to be with the preschool set, and the rest of us were seemingly spared. Matt left for a work trip out of town. It was March break in Halifax and there were lots of kid-friendly activities happening around the city. We hit up the museum, the science centre, and had play dates with friends. I was at the library with the girls and our friends one morning when I started to feel... funny. I knew instantly it was my turn with the stomach bug. I quickly headed home, calling my mom on the way to come over and watch the girls. By the time she arrived I was full-on sick, retching into a bucket from my bed when I wasn't running for the toilet. My mom slept the night on the couch, unable to leave me alone with the girls. The next morning, Matt woke up with the stomach bug, too, and had to drive home from New Brunswick, barf bag at the ready.

He rebounded quickly, but just when I thought I was coming around, the illness returned with a vengeance. Four days after the whole thing started, I was violently ill: I threw up twelve times in a row. I was unable to retain any fluids. We called my parents to come over late Sunday night, and shortly after 10:00 P.M. Matt helped me, barely able to stand, into the car. We were off to the emergency room with me vomiting along the way.

When I arrived, the nurses in triage couldn't even detect my blood pressure. Typically, things move pretty slowly at the ER but we arrived in triage at 10:18 P.M., I was registered by 10:32, and I was lying on a stretcher by 10:40, where the nurses were attempting, without success, to insert an IV line. There was a flurry of commotion. The stretcher was positioned at an incline so my legs were higher than my head to help raise my blood pressure. I was hooked up to a cardiac monitor. At 10:55 someone finally got the IV line into my weakened veins. They

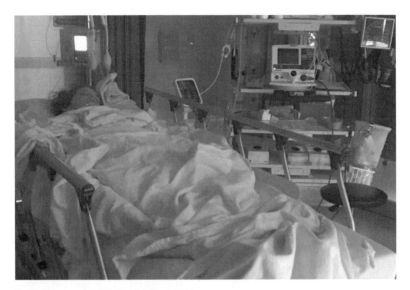

Heather's very rough night in the ER in March 2017.

started to hydrate me as quickly as possible with a large volume of fluid, using a pressure bag for rapid infusion, then repeated the same process over again. I was shaking from the cold, so they wrapped me in warm blankets. Within ten minutes my blood pressure finally began to rise. I felt completely disoriented and very uncomfortable, vaguely aware that I was moaning and hollering incomprehensibly.

"Are you in pain?" a nurse asked me.

"No," I muttered, my body tense, my respiratory rate increasing.

"Are you cold?"

"No," I denied, shivering profusely.

"Try to slow down your breathing," the nurse instructed. "Try to relax." Matt had been standing to the side, helplessly taking in the scene. He started trying to calm me down too.

I was panicking—anxious beyond my control. Two attempts at drawing blood failed. Half an hour later my respiratory rate started increasing again. I was given Ativan to calm me down. Eventually my veins gave up some blood for testing, and by midnight my blood pressure was finally stable.

Throughout the night, more fluids were pumped into me, along with Zofran, Tylenol, ibuprofen, an antibiotic called ceftriaxone (in case of bacterial infection), and Flagyl (another antibiotic). The blood work was repeated and then, just like that, I was discharged from my fourth emergency-room admission in the past twelve months.

Three days later I was still feeling very sick. Reluctantly, I returned to the emergency room, dehydrated again, and this time with abdominal pain. A set of X-rays showed distended gas-filled bowels, but no definite obstruction or perforation. The doctors wanted to admit me, but there was no bed available. I spent the night in a room that seemed to be an

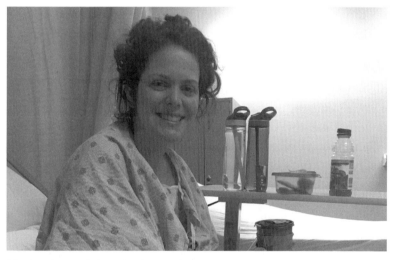

A few days after her stint in the ER in March 2017, Heather was admitted and spent a few days recovering on the eighth floor of the QEII.

offshoot of the emergency department, but at least this space was quiet and private, tucked away from the commotion of the emergency room. A flexible sigmoidoscopy was ordered the next day and I was knocked out for it. The scoped showed some mild narrowing of the bowel, but the summary report concluded: *There is no active disease. There is no active inflammation. Heather's Crohn's disease is not active at this point. Symptoms are most likely secondary to a viral infection and should settle with supportive management.*

When a room finally became available, I was moved to the eighth floor for two days of rest with plenty of fluids and electrolytes. It was very different from my usual hospital stay. There was no NG tube stuck up my nose, and I was allowed to eat and drink whatever I could tolerate. Matt delivered tea, juice, and toasted bagels from Tim Hortons, and grilled cheese sandwiches from our favourite diner. As long as I continued to improve, the doctor promised I'd be out of there in a few days.

On Sunday morning Matt took the kids to their friend's birthday party. The girls jumped around on the bouncy castle, twirled under the brightly coloured parachute, and ate lots of cake. Then they swung by the hospital to pick up their mother, as if it was just another weekend errand.

Ambulatory Care Clinic Letter
Gastroenterology Clinic, QEII Health Sciences Centre
October 30, 2017

Dear Elena:

I reviewed Heather in the clinic today. She is a very pleasant 35-year-old female who I have been following for Crohn's disease. At present, she is well in remission on Remicade 400 mg q.4 weeks. She is also on 6-MP 75 mg daily.

At this point, she is completely asymptomatic. I would recommend that she be vaccinated with the flu shot annually, as well she will need to be vaccinated for pneumococcus with both the Prevnar and the Pneumovax. I will leave those arrangements in your hands. [Regarding] routine maintenance, she will also need a flexible sigmoidoscopy with biopsies done. I will do that in the very near future. I have also reviewed her lab work which shows very slightly high protein. We will follow up with a protein electrophoresis. This may certainly be a paraprotein related to her treatment; however, I will follow up on this.

I will see her again at the time of flexible sigmoidoscopy and keep you informed of our findings.

Yours sincerely,
Dana Farina, MD, FRCPC
Attending Staff, Dept. of Med (Gastroenterology)

Seven months later, as fall rolled around, I was doing well. In October, we welcomed a rambunctious boxer puppy named Gabby to the family—as if we didn't already have enough on our plates. Because I'd had that scope done in the hospital in March that showed no active Crohn's disease, and because my health was in such a great place, when the scope that had been ordered by the surgeon the previous summer finally came up, I cancelled the appointment. I honestly thought there was no need for it, but Dr. Farina was not happy to hear this. Because no biopsies had been collected at that most recent scope, he wanted to schedule another one. I was agreeable, but also knew it would be months before I got another appointment. In the meantime, Matt and I took a marvellous kid-free trip to New York City, then to Toronto before the holidays, and later in the new year, back to NYC. Crohn's was far from my mind.

Another eight months flew by; it was now spring 2018. Somehow, I was still in good health. I was taking my 6-MP tablets every night before bed without any side effects. Every four weeks I'd visit the infusion clinic to receive my Remicade. It had been nine years since I'd started Remicade. By this point the treatment was far more standard. The clinic had expanded to three treatment rooms: one a private room with just one chair (and its own TV); the other rooms had four chairs each—big comfy brown leather recliners. It was still the same scenario, nurses bustling around, starting up IV lines, filling out paperwork at their desks, chatting with patients—I'd been there dozens and dozens of times, so they knew me well. The infusion still took a couple of hours and they checked my vitals every thirty minutes or so, with the medication administered slowly at first, increasing in speed as the appointment went on to make sure my body tolerated it with no issues or reactions, as there had been that fall afternoon on my birthday nine years earlier. The nurse then had slowed the infusion down and administered Benadryl through the IV line. Now I took Benadryl tablets preventatively with every infusion.

This time the nurses got my IV flowing, which sometimes took a few pokes because I had so much scar tissue built up from years of IV needles. I usually didn't feel a thing, likely because of nerve damage. It was infusion number 109 for me, and the process had become routine. I settled into the oversized chair in one of the bigger rooms, the same chair in the same room where I always sat—a creature of habit. I was deep into the book I was reading when I started to feel funny. I tried to shrug it off, thinking it was all in my head, because I couldn't quite figure out what was going on. Suddenly I realized that whatever it was, it wasn't right.

"Can someone come here?" I called out in a panic. I glanced over at the only other person in the room, another woman receiving treatment two chairs away. She sat up attentively. Cathy, the nurse in charge of me that day—coincidentally a neighbour on my street—appeared immediately.

"I feel funny," I told her. "I think something is wrong." She stopped the infusion instantly. I was short of breath and my heart was skipping beats; I had little palpitations in my chest. I realized I could be having an allergic reaction to the medication. I was terrified my throat was going to close up and I wouldn't be able to breathe. Then suddenly I got chills. Cathy methodically sprang into action, checking my vitals. My heart rate was increasing, and I was spiking a fever. I felt dizzy. A doctor was on call in the building for situations like this and Cathy called to have the doctor assess me. Cathy also phoned Matt to let him know what was happening. I was comforted that Cathy had been assigned to me that day; she knew our family and often chatted with the girls in our yard.

It didn't take long for Matt to get there from his nearby office; he rushed in, breathless. Benadryl was being administered through the IV along with hydrocortisone. I was given Tylenol to swallow. There was nothing to do but wait and see how my body responded. The on-call doctor recommended I recline the chair and lay back, but I felt really anxious in that position. I wanted to sit up with my feet grounded firmly on the floor. I realized the clinic was now empty—both the room next door that had had patients earlier, and room I was in. The other woman had quietly slipped by me once her own infusion finished.

The fast heart rate, dizziness, fever, and chills persisted, and my chest remained tight. Because my heart rate wouldn't come down and there was nothing more the clinic could offer, it was time to call 911. In just moments we heard the siren wail, the ambulance making its way to me through the city streets. The paramedics were kind, checking me over, but there wasn't much more they could offer than safe transportation to the emergency department. I was mortified as they loaded me onto a stretcher and rolled me through the lobby of the busy professional centre, right past the Starbucks. I prayed I didn't bump into anyone I knew.

We arrived to a packed emergency room around 5:30 P.M. Matt met us there. I started to feel a tingling sensation around my mouth. One of the paramedics had to wait with us in a long hallway lined with stretchers, unable to leave me until I was seen by a physician. I dozed on and off, the Benadryl making me sleepy. Finally, at 7:00 P.M., a doctor appeared at the side of my stretcher. There was still no room for me, so she consulted with me there in the hall. The symptoms had subsided, and I was feeling okay. Exhausted, but okay. The doctor said it was fine for me to head home, with instructions to keep taking Benadryl for a couple of days and follow up with my doctor.

I had to pause the Remicade infusions. Thankfully my Crohn's symptoms remained in check. With an allergy, the immune system overreacts to the allergen by producing antibodies. I needed a special blood test to check for those antibodies in my system.

If I turned out to be allergic, I would not be able to take Remicade again without the risk of another allergic-type reaction. But first we had to wait for the Remicade levels in my blood to drop. After a round of therapeutic drug monitoring (TDM)—the testing that measures the amount of drug left in the blood—the levels (at eleven) were too high to measure the antibody level.

At a follow-up appointment in July, Dr. Farina wrote me prescriptions for budesonide and prednisone in the event I developed symptoms while waiting for the results of the antibody test. I was to try the budesonide first; the prednisone was a last resort. The hope was that I would not need either one.

When he rechecked the TDM, the antibody levels came back negative, although the drug level was still not completely down to zero. Dr. Farina reviewed charts from the reaction again and decided it did not clearly sound like an allergic reaction; he wanted to get me back on Remicade. I was to be premedicated with IV Benadryl (at a higher dose than the tablets I'd been taking at my infusions) and hydrocortisone, and the infusion rate would be slower to prevent a reaction.

He went over the risks with me—including anaphylaxis—but believed the risk was acceptably low. Arrangements were made to restart my infusions in the next few weeks. He also wrote me a prescription for Ativan to help with any associated anxiety at the thought of another—potentially worse—reaction.

In the aftermath of dealing with the drug reaction, the appointment date for that scope finally arrived. It was scheduled for Anna's first day of grade primary. There was no way I was missing that milestone just to have an assessment of a disease that was currently in check. This time, I checked in with Dr. Farina's office before I cancelled the appointment. I explained I was feeling all right, and that I wouldn't be able to make the date scheduled for the scope. His office assured me these things happen—appointment dates don't always work out—and they'd put me back on the list.

I restarted the Remicade infusions that fall. To my relief, the infusion, and the two that followed, went very well. The infusion now took five hours. It was a s-l-o-w drip, with an additional half hour for the pre-medications. The IV Benadryl made me so drowsy that the rest of the day was a writeoff; I was useless. I wasn't allowed to drive home from the appointments, so I had to arrange to be dropped off and picked up. A small perk was that I now had access to the private room, perhaps to keep me calm or maybe to keep me separate from the other patients in case I had another reaction. I was just happy I didn't have to deal with anyone snoring or talking loudly. I had my own private TV so I could pick the shows I wanted to watch. Sometimes I tried to get work done or read; sometimes I mindlessly scrolled on my phone; mostly I slept. I took the Ativan for the first two appointments but didn't feel the need for it at the third appointment. I was also extending the time between appointments to six weeks rather than four.

Everything was going well until my appointment in January.

Not long after everything was set up and the IV was flowing with my pre-meds, I felt my lips start tingling. The nurse arrived and hung the bag with the Remicade; I had barely received a drop when my heart started pounding. Suddenly I couldn't catch my breath; after a quick check of my vitals the nurse said my blood pressure was rising. The nurse stopped the infusion and gave me more Benadryl; I also popped an Ativan. The symptoms dissipated, but it was clear my infusion was not proceeding.

Now we had a mystery; I'd never had this sensation outside of the Remicade infusion clinic. There was no difference in the premedications I'd received at the three previous appointments. I'd been fine without the Ativan at the last appointment. I started to wonder if it could have been a panic attack.

It was three weeks before I could get an appointment with Dr. Farina. It had been nine weeks since I'd had the medication and my bowels were starting to feel irritated. I agreed with the doctor that it was difficult to attribute the latest reaction to the Remicade given that the reaction occurred after I had received barely any of the medication. However, the symptoms of my heart pounding and increased blood pressure could very well be attributed to the steroids I was receiving as one of the premedication drugs. We decided to give the Remicade another go without the hydrocortisone. I'd have Benadryl and Tylenol and take the Ativan.

With my health stable—my definition of stable, dealing with the chronic abscesses and fistulas that were mostly at bay, sometimes flaring up—the rest of 2019 passed uneventfully, with still no sign of the appointment for that scope.

I had no issues at my next infusion. Eventually, after many more smooth appointments, I stopped taking the Ativan, continuing to bring it along with me "just in case." With Anna in the thick of grade one and Rosie at preschool, I was able to ramp up my freelance work, writing lifestyle articles for the newspaper and local magazines. We welcomed the new year in 2020 with a family trip to Mexico. It was one of those trips we couldn't really afford, but we did it anyway because we wanted a beach destination vacation so badly.

We returned home on February 2 with nothing but good memories—as opposed to the new year in 2016 when I'd ended up in the hospital with an obstruction, or the scary trip to the emergency room with severe dehydration from gastroenteritis in March 2017, or the drug reactions I dealt with going into 2019.

We'll be forever grateful we took that trip—because one month later the world shut down.

AMBASSADOR FOR THE CAUSE

"Heather Fegan is in the prime of her life, newly married to the man of her dreams and in a career that she loves. You'd never guess that from the age of fourteen Heather endured consistent periods of pain because of flare-ups caused by Crohn's disease..."

This is the voiceover to a news story I took part in during the fall of 2008 with Dr. Desmond Leddin, the head of digestive care and endoscopy at Dalhousie University, who had helped guide me to my first surgery.

There are scenes of Matt and me strolling down a city street outside our condo, making dinner in our kitchen, and flipping through our wedding album. In the interview I talk about my diagnosis and my journey, how I had travelled to Toronto for a dream-job interview during a major flare-up, and how from there I had started a new treatment that helped me feel well again. Dr. Leddin spoke to the medical side of the disease and the newer treatments available with biologic drugs like Remicade and Humira.

This was in the early fall of 2008; I was taking part in a media campaign to help educate Canadians about quality of life for people living with Crohn's disease. Along with filming the prepackaged news segment for TV, there was an article about me in the newspaper (the same paper where I would later become a regular columnist), and I participated in some on-air live interviews at various radio and TV stations around the city.

In addition to tirelessly conducting radio and TV interviews, I was also sitting on panels (in Halifax, Montreal, and Toronto) organized by the Crohn's and Colitis Foundation of Canada (CCFC) and speaking on behalf of young people with Crohn's disease.

But this wasn't the first time I had volunteered for the foundation. My volunteering had actually begun when I was first diagnosed. My mom and I started helping out at the registration table at the annual Heel 'n' Wheel-a-Thon fundraiser (now called the Gutsy Walk), eventually building our own team

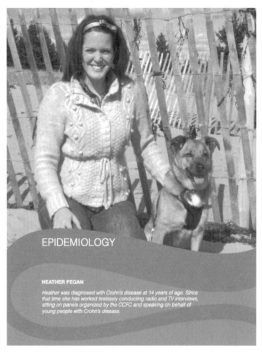

EPIDEMIOLOGY

HEATHER FEGAN

Heather was diagnosed with Crohn's disease at 14 years of age. Since that time she has worked tirelessly conducting radio and TV interviews, sitting on panels organized by the CCFC and speaking on behalf of young people with Crohn's disease.

Heather has volunteered in numerous roles with Crohn's and Colitis Canada over the years in an effort to help raise awareness and funding for research. Here she's seen in a page from the *2012 Impact of IBD* report.

to participate in the walk/run/roll along the waterfront, then actually running the whole event—along with the group of other passionate volunteers, of course.

I helped run a popular annual barbecue with the help of friends who volunteered with me, and in later years I helped my sister organize "All That Glitters" galas—glitzy and glamorous affairs raising thousands and thousands of dollars. Eventually, I stepped into the role of president of the Halifax chapter of the CCFC.

While it wasn't a support group, it was a supportive group. We met once a month in a community space. The faces became very familiar over the years, and we were all connected through Crohn's—either our own or affecting someone we loved. Supported by the regional director of the foundation, we worked hard to increase the profile of IBD and to raise money toward finding a cure. We organized awareness events and educational meetings, and did lots of fundraising, commiserating, celebrating, and connecting. When I started a family my volunteering moved to the back burner, but I suspect I'll return to it at some point.

In the fall of 2011, I received a very special honour. November is Crohn's and Colitis Awareness month—a time when the foundation steps up its media coverage, launching a campaign designed to raise awareness of IBD and funds for research. There are regional and national conferences, many of which I have attended. In 2011, I was awarded the title of the "Gutsiest Canadian in the Maritimes" by the foundation (which later became Crohn's and Colitis Canada). In addition to receiving a fun prize package, I and the other "gutsiest Canadians" from across the country were profiled in *The Journal*, the foundation's publication:

Heather is being celebrated for her courage in facing inflammatory bowel disease (IBD) and for her outstanding work to make a difference in her community and in the lives of others. Since being diagnosed with Crohn's disease at the age of fourteen, Heather has worked tirelessly to support the IBD community. As a role model to many IBD patients, Heather speaks openly about her illness and has volunteered much of her time to raising funds and awareness to help find a cure. Heather demonstrates a tremendous amount of confidence, courage and strength and is an inspiration to her family and friends. This Gutsy Canadian won't let anything stop her from reaching her goals and will help as many others along the way as she can.

I accepted the award at the National Symposium Conference in Halifax during that year's awareness month, complete with an acceptance speech to share my story.

SIX STEPS FOR SELF-ADVOCACY

Whether you're facing a new diagnosis of Crohn's disease or ulcerative colitis, or you're a seasoned veteran with years of experience with IBD, the experts I spoke with suggest six important steps when it comes to self-advocacy:

Know your illness

"My best advice is for patients to know their disease," says registered IBD nurse practitioner Barbara Currie. "Know where it is, know the treatments they've been on, what worked, what didn't." Currie says it's important that patients can communicate this kind of information, including what they think is going on.

"At the end of the day, people need to understand…what makes it better, what makes it worse, what their responses to treatments are. …We really need to work together as a team to manage the life of a person living with a lifelong chronic disease."

Dr. Jennifer Jones, team lead of the NSCIBD program at the QEII Health Sciences Centre, says one of the problems in communicating what's happening with your illness is a lack of integration in health information systems. "Nothing is connected. Even if they just allowed systems to talk to each other…[but] they don't. It's a big problem."

Jones does offer one suggestion for patients—that they put together a disease-related summary that they can always keep with them. "[Then] when they are encountering people in the emergency room or in their family physician's office or another specialist's office, they have it there at their fingertips, and when they're flaring or distraught, they don't have to then try to focus and pull this information to the forefront." Jones also suggests patients keep phone numbers for their care providers at hand.

Communicate honestly

Following regimens and staying committed to treatment plans can be hard.

"One of the things I say to my patients is, 'How often do you forget to take your medicine?' Not, 'Do you forget?' because we all forget and we're human," explains Currie. "And it's okay to tell me that you've forgotten, because I need up-to-date information if I'm going to interpret your symptoms and your lab reports and your diagnostic tests. If you haven't been taking your medication for six months, I need to know that. We can still work together and try to improve your health moving forward."

Currie says patients should not be afraid to tell their clinicians that they aren't taking a medication, whether it's because they can't afford it, it makes them sick, or they're afraid to take it. "We can help address some of those concerns and figure out ways around them," Currie says, noting that many people carry a lot of guilt and self-blame when they don't take a medication. "If I was taking a medicine every day that made me sick, I probably wouldn't want to take it either. We have to meet patients where they're at," she says, "so how are we going to work together moving forward to monitor the Crohn's or the ulcerative colitis, and what will we do if they have a significant flare? I think sometimes patients just need to know that there's a plan if things change drastically."

Currie says sometimes people just need a drug holiday, or they just want to forget about their IBD. "But the challenge is oftentimes when we do that, the patient flares. They need to know that there's a way back. …I say be your advocate, be honest, be truthful to your clinician because we're working together to optimize the patient's health."

Accept responsibility for your health

In addition to understanding their disease and communicating honestly to their healthcare providers, patients must accept responsibility for their own health. "Getting their blood work done, doing their stool testing if the clinician asked them to, …coming for their scopes when booked, and making their appointments," says Currie, "that's all part of being an adult and managing your health."

Currie says the clinic's job is to work within the patient's expectations and acceptance of treatment that's being offered to them. "My job is to provide the most expert opinion on a management strategy for somebody's inflammatory bowel disease. And their responsibility is to decide if they want to accept that recommendation. At the end of the day, that's how I see the equation," she says. "We're not in the business of forcing people to do anything; we're in the business of making a recommendation for the most efficacious plan to treat inflammatory bowel disease that works for the patients…and it's their job to decide if that's something they want."

Currie points out that the onus is on patients to respond to changes in their symptoms because they know themselves best. The clinician only knows what the patient is telling them. "We can do objective markers of inflammation, we can do scopes, we can do all kinds of things, but the patient's living with it every day, so they know if it's a one-off day or more than that," she says.

Another important element to accepting responsibility is advocating to be seen when you need to be seen.

"If you're lucky enough to have access to a helpline, make use of it," says Dr. Jones. "Don't downplay your symptoms and assume that they're going to pass. Pick up the phone and call the line because that's what it's there for." She says if you're not fortunate enough to have access to a helpline, it's important to advocate to ensure that your primary care doctor understands that you may be experiencing a flare-up so they can suggest what the next steps should be.

There are some barriers, however, that patients can't advocate through. If you don't have a primary care doctor, you have no one to advocate to.

"In collaboration with Crohn's and Colitis Canada's PACE network we are implementing an externally facing nurse navigational role to overcome access inequity for marginalized populations," says Jones. An initiative of Crohn's and Colitis Canada, the Promoting Access and Care through Centres of Excellence (PACE) program brings together leading IBD centres from across the country to drive changes in the public healthcare system.

"This is happening across the country in multiple provinces, and we're specifically going to be researching that role for implementation of evidence-based care pathways to improve access to that type of care for patients. One of the purposes of this navigational role is to try to overcome some of those barriers and work with communities on solutions to overcome them."

Seek reliable resources

In keeping with learning about and understanding your disease, Currie stresses the importance of using reliable resources in the quest for knowledge.

"Crohn's and Colitis Canada is a great resource for information," she says. "Somebody's blog is not a good source of reliable scientific information about inflammatory bowel disease."

She acknowledges that Facebook groups for people with Crohn's and colitis can be very helpful in terms of normalizing feelings related to stressful situations and procedures. "Those kinds of groups can be very supportive, but you have to make sure that it's not just people who are dissatisfied," she says, "because that's a slippery slope. Knowing where to get good information is important."

Access peer support

"Don't be alone," says Dr. Michael Vallis, a registered health psychologist whose practice focusses on people with chronic diseases. Vallis suggests patients seek out support groups, and he points to organizations like Crohn's and Colitis Canada as well as the Ostomy Canada Society. "Find a voice, chat rooms, Facebook—try to recognize that you're not alone."

Vallis says the symptoms of IBD can be socially isolating. "I believe that anything that helps to normalize the experience, that could really promote a better understanding and acceptance of those emotional issues, that social component of it, is actually really important."

Crohn's and Colitis Canada has local chapters in every province across the country. While not official "support groups," they offer supportive places where people can connect with their local IBD community. They also offer the opportunity to volunteer and to support people living with IBD which, for many, is an important way of giving back.

Cultivate support systems

Medical appointments can be stressful; it can help to bring someone with you who can act as a second set of ears and who can advocate on your behalf. "Sometimes that's helpful, particularly at times when you're not feeling well or you're in a flare and your mind is a bit scrambled," says Barbara Currie. "It's good to have somebody else who can say, 'Yeah, that's what your clinician said,' or, 'No, I think they may have said this.'"

MY STORY:
CROHN'S IN THE TIME OF
COVID-19 AND BEYOND
(2020–2023)

Like most people, my family and I had never anticipated a pandemic in our lifetime, but there we were, living history in 2020 as the Covid-19 virus spread around the world. We'd recently returned from Mexico and friends were cancelling their March break family vacations. We cancelled a local one-night hotel stay we'd planned to enjoy after a day of skiing; being in a communal environment just didn't feel like the right thing to do. When we heard that the NBA basketball league was shutting down, we knew things were getting serious.

Luckily, I'd had a Remicade infusion right before everything began to shut down. The school's March break was extended for two weeks to "flatten the curve," so we hunkered down as a family, playing games, watching movies, baking, roaming the neighbourhood on daily walks, meeting with friends for virtual drinks—not yet consumed with Zoom fatigue. At first, we were all-in for all the at-home activities we could come up with. Then school didn't reopen. Matt and I were lucky to be able to split the day while working from home. We each got half a day in the home office and half a day with the kids, then caught up on work in the evenings after the kids were in bed—not that I had a lot to do, given that freelance work was drying up as publications paused their presses.

For five weeks I didn't shop anywhere (Matt was the designated household shopper) or go anywhere, aside from walking in the neighbourhood, dropping goodies off on a friend's doorstep, and waving to my parents from their front lawn. I drove the car twice in a month.

But then it was time for my next infusion. It was like being granted a pass. I could get out of the house—out of the neighbourhood. I'd see other people, catch up with some lovely women, get closer than six feet to them—and spend five hours there. The concern, though, was that the very medication I was going to receive to keep me healthy, Crohn's-wise, was going to leave me at risk, infection-wise.

While as citizens we'd all been washing our hands, social-distancing, self-isolating, and doing what we could to stay healthy and keep our immune systems in check, I was heading out to actively wear mine down. The whole point of the drug was to suppress my immune system along with the other immunosuppressant, 6-MP, that I took daily. Remicade and 6-MP are used to treat a number of autoimmune diseases, but they lower the body's ability to fight infections. Crohn's caused my body to attack its healthy cells, mainly in the GI tract, resulting in inflammation—at times, debilitating inflammation. The medications suppressed the immune system by blocking that overactive attacking of the GI tract.

The pandemic introduced a new complication. The Public Health Agency of Canada deemed having a compromised immune system a moderate risk for infection and serious complications of Covid-19. The advice for those at medium-risk because of IBD and immunosuppressive drugs was to avoid in-person meetings, work from home, use virtual technology, and use the services designed to help vulnerable people avoid contact with others, such as early shopping hours at the grocery store. We had pre-emptively stalked up on everything we'd need for the next little while so we could avoid going out.

I set out for my appointment, driving through eerily empty city streets. When I arrived at the usually bustling professional building that held the clinic, I found a ghost town. I was greeted by silence. There was no missing the memo—signs were plastered everywhere telling people not to enter and to stay home if they had any symptoms or had been travelling. Only those with appointments should be in the building.

I knocked on the clinic door that had never been locked before, waiting to be let in. Before allowing me in, the nurse asked a million questions about symptoms, travel, and potential exposure and took my temperature. All was good and I was allowed to enter. As I settled into my seat the nurse noticed some welts on my neck—before I even started receiving the drug. They were totally due to stress. I was nervous about being there! I had Ativan with me "just in case," so before long, I was feeling cool as a cucumber.

After more than thirty days at home with the kids, I was happy to settle in with a book to pass the time. I spent the morning by myself in the small private room. At lunchtime someone else needed the room so I was moved into one of the two main treatment rooms. It holds four chairs, but two of them were out of bounds. An elderly lady came in, and she and I were seated at opposite ends of the room to receive our treatments. The other treatment room had three of five chairs filled with patients; it was a very quiet day in the clinic.

The space looked like the clinic was either just moving in or about to move out. Everything had been packed up to minimize the number of things people might touch. Three nurses I knew well were working. They were wearing gloves and masks, but otherwise it was business as usual for them—they continued

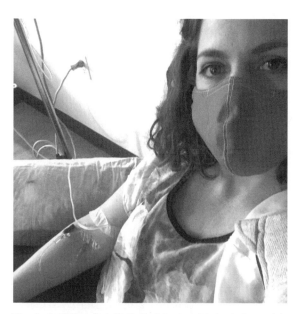

When the Covid-19 pandemic hit, Heather's Remicade infusions took on a whole new set of protocols designed to limit potential exposure to Covid-19. This photo was taken in November 2020.

to leave their homes and go to work every day. I'm sure they hoped their patients were doing all the right things to limit their exposure to Covid-19, but these nurses were there for us no matter what. Fortunately, it's the kind of clinic where anyone with any kind of infection would be prevented from receiving treatment because of the harm it could do, so the risk of catching something there was low at any time.

Everything felt very clean. Every time someone used the washroom, the staff went straight in to wipe everything down. Only nurses were opening door handles. There was a lot of handwashing going on and there were bottles of hand sanitizer all around.

I was still offered a drink—coffee, tea, water, or juice, only this time the coffee came in a disposable cup. I was also still offered a snack but wasn't allowed to physically pick it out of the basket myself. I picked what I wanted and the nurse handed it over. They also weren't allowed to hand out blankets or pillows, so I was freezing all day—it feels cold having fluids pumped into you. The nurses would normally check my vitals every twenty to thirty minutes to make sure everything was fine. They'd start the infusion slowly and bump it up in phases over the five hours until it was flowing at max. But this time, to limit physical contact, they checked my vitals only at the start and at the end of the infusion and just asked me to let them know if I felt odd.

Before I left, the nurse handed me a letter permitting me to venture out for my next treatment should the lockdown get even tighter. That brought a grim reality to the situation unfolding all around us—the unknown variables Covid-19 was inflicting. No matter what was to come, I'd still need this treatment—in fact, more than ever—to keep my health in check so I didn't wind up in an over-taxed hospital, alone, during a flare-up.

With all the lockdowns, isolations, and the cancelled appointments and surgeries we were hearing about on the news, I knew I wasn't going to get that scope I was still waiting for anytime soon. It was interesting to be an immunocompromised person during this time, but it didn't impact me negatively. We continued taking the same precautions everyone else was taking to avoid the virus. As things started opening up and we were able to slowly expand our social circles, we were cautious but still lived our lives, always following the rules.

Nova Scotia's approach to the pandemic was cautious, and our lockdowns, border closures, and strict quarantine rules worked—until they didn't. Early on, people worked together to keep others safe, allowing us to live with very low rates of Covid-19. Our little province, then part of the Atlantic Bubble, garnered coverage in the *New York Times*. Journalist Stephanie Nolen wrote: "We gather without fear. Life is unfolding much as it did a year ago. This magical, virus-free world is just one long day's drive away from the Empire State Building—in a parallel dimension called Nova Scotia." This came at an expense, of course; the economy suffered, quarantining was difficult for those who had to do it, social interactions and relationships were affected, and seniors in nursing care were segregated from their loved ones, many dying in isolation. But it meant there was a low threat of the virus in the general population, so in return most of us had freedom. And those of us who were more vulnerable were safer, which was reassuring.

Thankfully, 2020 was a quiet year in terms of my health, but as the calendar ticked over to 2021, I began to feel unwell again. For weeks I had abdominal pain and obstruction-like symptoms that never escalated but also wouldn't go away. Christmas break had been extended for the kids because of another wave of Covid-19. I helped facilitate online learning, working alongside the kids by day and lying on the couch binge-watching *Bridgerton* by night. I never fully enjoyed the show because pains were stabbing in my abdomen. Fever and chills were intermittent, but PCR tests for Covid-19 always came up negative. I finally got an appointment with my family doctor toward the end of January, who referred me to the emergency room to see if we could get to the bottom of what was going on and get me some help with hydration.

A trip to the emergency room is never a good time on an ordinary day, but if you think that experience can't get worse—layer a pandemic on top of it.

The department was almost at capacity the evening I arrived. Someone was stationed at the door to screen arrivals, asking the typical Covid-related questions. I let them know I'd had a negative PCR test a couple of days earlier, with no fever since before the test. They said Matt could come in and wait with me, but if any other patients came in, he'd have to leave. We were handed medical masks and ushered to a waiting area. The place was packed, and after avoiding crowds for so long, it felt wrong—especially to be stuck in this kind of crowd, with sick people all around. I pleaded with Matt to leave; we didn't *both* need to sit there and be exposed. Eventually they called me up to triage. The nurse, who looked like she was run ragged, was curt, asking for my information and taking my vitals. I started to explain my symptoms, my Crohn's history, describing how the past few weeks had played out.

"You've had a fever?" she snapped.

"Yes, but I'm negative for Covid," I replied. "I told them at the door."

"That test was days ago," she snapped again, then proceeded to make a big show of donning extra PPE, exasperatedly wiping clean all the equipment she'd used on me.

"This is my Crohn's," I tried to explain.

"It's going to be a ten to twelve hour wait," she informed me, as if it were my fault. "And you'll have to wait over there for Covid screening." She pointed to one half of the waiting room, an area designated for Covid-symptomatic patients. I made my way back to Matt and explained the situation to him through tears. There weren't even any seats left. I'd be hanging out with a crowd of sick people for ten to twelve hours, sitting on the floor. There was no possible way.

We were out of there.

Gastroenterology Clinic
QEII Health Sciences Centre
February 03, 2021

Dear Elena:

I reviewed Heather by phone today. She is a very pleasant 38-year-old female who I have been following for Crohn's disease. Her involvement has always been at the ileorectal anastomosis. She had been feeling really well through 2020; however, on January 2, 2021, she started to develop some obstructive-like symptoms. She was alternating between diarrhea and constipation. She would have quite significant bloating with this, to the point where she would be significantly distended and have sharp epigastric pains.

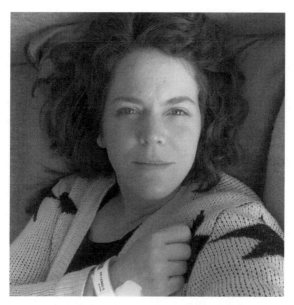

A groggy looking Heather recovers from her February 2021 sigmoidoscopy.

She did have a sinus infection midway through this, but did not take antibiotics. She was having difficulties with hydration and did go to the emergency [room]; however, did not wait at that time due to numerous factors.

She received a dose of Remicade last Thursday and her symptoms are now starting to improve. As of today, she is feeling back to her normal. She is currently on Remicade q.6 weeks.

She did not start prednisone during this episode.

At this point, I think the best thing to do is to reassess her disease. We do have recent blood work which did show a high CRP, as well as a high ferritin, which again would go along with an inflammatory process.

I will book her for a sigmoidoscopy in the next week or so and keep you informed of our findings.

Yours sincerely,
Dana Farina, MD, FRCPC
Attending Staff, Dept. of Med (Gastroenterology)

Thankfully my symptoms didn't advance after leaving the emergency department. The time came for my Remicade infusion, which helped matters. In early February I had a virtual appointment with my GI doctor, who decided we should reassess my disease. My C-reactive protein (CRP) level (a marker indicating inflammation in the body) was at 54. A normal level is 0.3 mg/dL; 1 to 10 mg/dL is considered moderate elevation, and anything over 10 is considered high. It was finally time to get serious about that scope.

A week and a half later, I had the procedure. I was sedated for the sigmoidoscopy, thankfully, and don't remember a thing. The test showed severe disease activity in the rectum, friability of surrounding tissue, erosions, and ulcers. The doctors had difficulty manoeuvring the scope; the area was significantly inflamed, but the results were similar to those from previous exams, as noted in the final report.

Nevertheless, I continued to improve and felt mostly well through the spring. Following a virtual follow-up with Dr. Farina in April he reported:

> At present, she is in remission on Remicade q.6 weeks. She is feeling well overall. She did have a recent flare earlier in the year; however, things settled down after her Remicade infusion. She does have intermittent lower abdominal discomfort which feels similar to her kidney stones. It is my understanding that you have organized a renal ultrasound and that is likely still pending.
>
> At this point, I will see her again in six months' time. I have not made any changes to her current management. I have discussed the Covid-19 vaccines with her and certainly gone over the pros and cons, but the overall recommendation would certainly be for her to undergo vaccination when she is offered, also to not be overly concerned by the timing in regard to the vaccine with her Remicade and if possible, if she receives the Pfizer or Moderna, it should be given at initially studied intervals as opposed to a prolonged duration between doses.
>
> I will see her again in six months' time and keep you informed of our findings.
>
> Dana Farina, MD, FRCPC
> Attending Staff, Dept. of Med (Gastroenterology)

Dr. Farina had recommended I receive the Covid-19 vaccine at "initially studied intervals," meaning with doses scheduled at the intervals that had been recommended in the early studies. That was twenty-one or twenty-eight days apart, depending on the vaccine, for which two initial doses were required in order to be fully vaccinated. But there was a problem. Nova Scotia was rolling out a vaccine program based on age as a primary risk factor, meaning the oldest of the population had first access to the vaccine, rolling out to lower age groups from there. The time between the first and second vaccinations would be prolonged to allow for the older group to be fully vaccinated first. Unfortunately, there was no exception to this rule, despite what the science said about people on immuno-suppressive therapies requiring timely access to the second dose of vaccines.

A study published in the UK observed that a substantial number of people with IBD did not mount an adequate antibody response after the first dose. Most, however, had an adequate antibody response after receiving their second vaccine dose, regardless of what medications they were taking. So that meant that because of the immunosuppressive medications I was on, my body wouldn't be able to mount an adequate anti-SARS-CoV-2 antibody response after just one dose.

Other provinces had allowed those in high-risk categories (I was considered high-risk because of the immunosuppressives) to schedule priority vaccines. Nova Scotia hadn't budged on this, sticking rigidly to an age-based approach with no room for risk assessment.

There was advocacy for such change on a national level. A Covid-19 and inflammatory bowel disease task force was formed by Crohn's and Colitis Canada and led by gastroenter-ologists, epidemiologists, infectious disease and IBD experts, patient representatives, and community leaders. The task force called on the National Advisory Committee on Immunization (NACI) to include IBD patients on immunosuppression ther-apies on the list of exceptions for extended dosing intervals.

Given that Nova Scotia had nearly twelve thousand people living with IBD, many requiring immunosuppressive therapy, the need for policy change in Nova Scotia was urgent. Several thousand Nova Scotians would benefit from a timely dose of the second vaccine.

I set to work writing an op-ed for one of the local news networks about the issue. I also wrote directly to the chief medical officer of health, Dr. Robert Strang.

from: Fegan, Heather
to: Strang, Robert
date: May 20, 2021, 5:21 PM
subject: Re: vaccine administration for the immunosuppressed

Dr. Strang,

I am calling on the Nova Scotia Government to immediately implement change in Nova Scotia on the timing of the second dose of the Covid-19 vaccine for the subgroup of people that require it.

Other provinces such as Ontario have protocols for vulnerable groups such as those at high risk, including individuals on immunosuppressive therapies.

If those on immunosuppressives don't get the second vaccine in a timely interval we won't mount an adequate anti-SARS-CoV-2 antibody response with just one dose because of these immunosuppressive medications.

Please listen to science. If you ignore this, then you're ignoring science.

This affects thousands of Nova Scotians, especially considering Nova Scotia has the highest incidence of Crohn's disease and colitis in the world, not to mention other individuals on immunosuppressive drugs for managing other conditions.

Several thousand Nova Scotians will benefit from a timely dose of the second vaccine.

And several thousand first doses will be wasted otherwise.

Vaccinate us properly. Let us help reach 85 percent of the population vaccinated. Don't leave us exposed.

Please take a look at my opinion piece published in the Saltwire News Network this week.

I have posted it below for your attention.

Thank you for taking this into consideration.

Sincerely,
Heather

from: Strang, Robert
to: Fegan, Heather
date: May 20, 2021, 11:43 PM
subject: Re: vaccine administration for the immunosuppressed

Dear Ms. Fegan,

Thank you for your e-mail and we are looking at this information as we develop our 2nd vaccine dose plan.

Sincerely,
Dr. Robert Strang
Chief Medical Officer of Health
Department of Health and Wellness

from: Fegan, Heather
to: Strang, Robert
date: May 24, 2021, 10:03 PM
subject: Re: vaccine administration for the
immunosuppressed

Dr. Strang,

Thank you so much for your reply—I can only imagine how inundated you are on a daily basis and I appreciate you taking the time to respond.

In the press conference on Friday, you stated there is good support that the 105-day interval between vaccines is creating an even better immune response. Of course, this does not apply to everyone. Other provinces have implemented change. So can Nova Scotia. We need to let the ones who need a more timely second dose go first.

I am left not knowing if I should postpone my scheduled vaccine appointment on Wednesday in hopes the protocol changes and rebook when/if I have a chance at getting the second dose— and the proper antibody response—in a timely interval.

Thanks for your time,
Heather

from: Strang, Robert
to: Fegan, Heather
date: Jun 6, 2021, 9:38 PM
subject: Re: vaccine administration for the immunosuppressed

Dear Ms. Fegan,

Thank you for your email.

Nova Scotia's 1st dose vaccine roll-out has been primarily age-based. That strategy has allowed us to be highly efficient with vaccination and ahead of our expected schedule. Our 2nd dose roll-out is well under way and mirrors our 1st dose roll-out with age as the primary risk factor. Nova Scotians are being invited to move their 2nd dose appointments up in batches that will retain the sequence of our roll-out but compress the interval between doses for all Nova Scotians. With our expected supply, this strategy should allow everyone to move their 2nd dose appointment up by 2–4 weeks each, with all Nova Scotians having two doses of vaccine by September.

We thank all Nova Scotians for continuing to follow the appropriate public health protocols as we build our provincial immunity levels.

Sincerely,
Dr. Robert Strang
Chief Medical Officer of Health
Department of Health and Wellness

I wasn't getting anywhere with my advocacy. Even by inviting Nova Scotians to move their second dose appointment up by two to four weeks each, my second dose, at best, would be eight to ten weeks too late and I'd have lost the opportunity to mount the adequate antibodies, as the evidence showed.

I did manage to help one person. I received a note from a friend who had shared one of my Facebook posts about the issue. A friend of hers hadn't known she was eligible for the vaccine in her province, but she looked into it after seeing my post and was able to receive the vaccine right away.

In the end, I went around the system. I managed to find a pharmacist who was willing to help me out. He was a contact of Matt's, and Matt dropped into his pharmacy one day to talk to him about the problem. The pharmacist had a few extra doses and said if I came in there and then, I could have one. I got my second vaccine exactly three weeks after my first.

We had another great summer in 2021. I kept busy with writing contracts. We went camping and we were hiking at least every other weekend, if not more, thanks to a family hiking column I was writing for the newspaper. I was in a running club with some of my girlfriends; two of us ran in our first (virtual) 5K fundraiser run. On our fifteen-year wedding anniversary, Matt and I took the kids to Cape Breton for a few days, back to the scene of our proposal on the Cabot Trail. We made our annual trek to Prince Edward Island to play tourists and bum around the beaches.

Throughout the summer, the lower abdominal discomfort I was experiencing continued to come and go; it was more like an ache than the sharp pains I was used to. I noticed it seemed to relate to my menstrual cycle and wondered if there was a connection. By that fall, I was doing that balancing act again; sometimes I was well, sometimes I was not. I had a new pain in my upper abdomen. I had frequent obstruction-like symptoms: sharp pains, bloating, distension, and being unable to pass anything. These symptoms would come on and last for most of the day and night, and I'd wake up feeling okay the next day. Sometimes the pain would radiate up into my arms and shoulder. I started tracking my health on paper and noted I felt sick more days than I felt well.

In mid-November, seven months from my last follow-up, I had another virtual appointment with Dr. Farina. We talked about my recent symptoms, and he thought it would be reasonable to schedule an ultrasound of the pelvis to look for any signs of lesions which could be compressing on my bowels, as well as to look at my gallbladder. I was at risk for gallstones, given my history of IBD. It might explain the "attacking" symptoms and pain that was radiating into my shoulder. In the interim, my doctor also thought it would be reasonable to increase my Remicade to a q.4 week interval. I'd been on that dose before. We'd been trying to prolong the time between infusions, which was successful for a while, but maybe not so much anymore.

I was now awaiting two ultrasounds—one abdominal scan ordered by my family doctor for the upper gastric pain, and a pelvic scan to investigate the new symptoms. The appointment for the abdominal scan, ordered back in April, finally came up in mid-December. The results were "unremarkable." My pancreas, gallbladder, and kidneys all looked great; my spleen was slightly on the larger side. My family doctor phoned to talk to me about preventing fatty liver disease by reducing alcohol consumption and limiting carbs and increasing my intake of leafy greens, other veggies and fruit, and protein. I can't eat leafy greens as a rule, but I vowed to get more pulped-up spinach into my smoothies.

By January, the pains seemed to mostly resolve. They'd flare up just before my Remicade infusion, which was now randomly synced up to my menstrual cycle, then settle within days of treatment. I was grateful the appointments were now only four weeks apart.

Then came February 6, 2022.

It was set to be a busy Sunday. We started the day early with showers for the kids, everyone's hair washed and styled, and fresh, clean clothes. Friends were coming for coffee as a very belated Christmas get-together (they'd had the virus over the holidays, which had scuttled our plans). Then we'd be off to gymnastics, a play date, and then dinner with my parents. We all took Covid rapid tests to be on the safe side because we'd be seeing so many people throughout the day, including the grandparents. Then, I busied myself prepping for our guests. You can imagine my shock and dismay when I glanced at the four Covid-19 tests on the kitchen counter fifteen minutes later and saw three brightly positive results—only Matt's test was negative—and we were all totally symptom-free. We swiftly cancelled all our plans and shared the news with close friends and family.

"You'll never believe this!" I texted my friends in the group chat, sharing a photo of the tests, which I'd repeated to be sure. That evening, when I made Matt test again, his showed faintly positive as well. I'd barely left our street in recent days, but the girls had been in school and Matt had been to some meetings. Covid-19 was everywhere, so who knew where it came from? Ironically, the girls had just received their second dose of the vaccine three days earlier. Maybe we'd picked it up in line at the children's hospital in some weird twist of fate.

By bedtime, I had all the symptoms of a full-on head cold with a low-grade fever. Fortunately, the kids experienced nothing more than a few days with stuffy noses. Matt got by with a brutal head cold, working all the while. I, however, cycled through many symptoms. One day I was stuffed up, the next day I had a sore throat, the next day a cough, head-aches, and high fevers with hot flashes and chills. By day, I was in shorts and a tank top, sweating in front of a fan, then wrapped in layers of blankets, shivering, by night. I had to delay my Remicade infusion by a week, since I was scheduled to go during our quarantine. I obsessively checked my oxygen levels with the 02 monitor Public Health had sent over after I reported online that we had Covid-19 and I was immuno-compromised. A nurse called a couple of times to check in, but unless I got worse or was struggling to breathe, there was nothing to do.

The kids ruled the roost. We piled snacks onto the kitchen counter and they were practically on their own. Friends and family dropped off medicine, meals, treats, and activities for the kids. Thankfully the Olympics were on television, so we had sports playing in a constant stream. We themed the week with sports movies, including *Cool Runnings* and *Space Jam*. I had to write a feature magazine article—so I wrote it from my bed. By the end of the week, arts and crafts supplies were scattered everywhere, puzzles and toys covering the floors. Then, as fast as it came, Covid-19 left. Our seven-day quarantine was bookended with snowstorms and school cancellations, so by the end of it we'd been isolated at home for eleven days. On day eight, I spiked a fever once again, but by day ten I had been twenty-four hours fever-free. We cleaned up the house, feeling hungover from a party we hadn't even had.

Unfortunately, the fevers I experienced exacerbated things with my Crohn's. Two days after recovering from Covid, I was able to have my infusion. My blood work taken at that appointment showed my CRP at eighty-four, the highest it had been in a long time, indicating I had very significant inflammation in my body. Old fistulas and abscesses flared up, causing me a lot of discomfort. I was reacquainted with my old friend Cipro, the antibiotic that Dr. Farina wanted to pair with Flagyl, the antibiotic I didn't like. He let me start off with Cipro alone but instructed me to add the second antibiotic if I didn't improve. Thankfully, the two-week course of Cipro helped make me feel better. While I was still awaiting the abdominal ultrasound, the doctor scheduled a gastroscopy (where a camera goes down your throat) to check out my small bowel and investigate the upper abdominal pains I'd been experiencing. I was able to have the procedure in March, under sedation, and thankfully everything looked healthy. The doctor took some biopsies to check for H. pylori (a bacterial infection that affects the stomach) and celiac disease (a digestive disorder in which the small intestine is damaged by gluten), both of which came back negative. He said we'd have a follow-up once I'd had the pelvic ultrasound.

Two months later, near the end of May, I shot up in bed late at night from a dead sleep. In a panic, I ran down to the kitchen and shuffled through the stack of paperwork shoved in the junk drawer. There it was—a letter from the Nova Scotia Health Authority with my ultrasound appointment time. When the appointment notice had arrived weeks before, I'd shoved the letter into the pile of mail to deal with later.

My appointment had been that morning at 10:00 A.M. I had missed it, yet somehow, deep in my sleep, my mind had registered it. I had never done anything like that in my life. I'd never missed an appointment, a procedure, even a deadline. Sure, I was busy organizing a book festival, which was coming up at the beginning of June, as well as writing my own book and handling all the things that come along with having two active kids, including volunteering as the president of the parent-teacher association. But I felt like a complete idiot. Perhaps because I was feeling well the test hadn't been on my radar. That morning I called the clinic and was put back on the waitlist. I'd already waited six months.

Over the summer I kept putting myself on week-long courses of Cipro because my symptoms were recurring. It would help, I'd come off the antibiotic, and things would flare up. At an appointment in August, Dr. Farina pulled a colorectal surgeon into the room for a quick impromptu consultation. Given my history and the results of my scopes, she thought I was a sitting duck for infection or a bowel obstruction and likely needed a proctectomy to remove the rest of the large bowel including the rectum—a difficult surgery that would leave me with a permanent ostomy. I promptly agreed to try Flagyl again.

I was getting desperate. As expected, it was a bad experience—worse than before. It made me dizzy, gave me a terrible metallic taste in my mouth, increased my sensitivity to smell, and I couldn't drink any alcohol while taking it, which was, well, fine—but no fun.

On the morning of my Remicade infusion at the end of August I woke up with thrush lesions (essentially a yeast infection) all over my tongue and in my mouth, and three blistering cold sores on my lips—side effects from the Flagyl. I arrived at the infusion clinic where they said they had to talk with my doctor before proceeding, given the state I was in. I sat there for two hours while they waited for confirmation from the GI clinic. No, I could not receive my infusion with these infections. I'd need to delay the Remicade. Now the nasty antibiotic was preventing me from taking my biologic, which was going to cause even bigger problems. After a three-week course, not only was it not making me feel any better—it was making me worse. I decided it wasn't worth the trouble, and with the blessing of Dr. Farina I stopped taking it. But I stayed on the Cipro. As soon as the infections cleared, with the help of another antiviral medication and a mouth rinse, I was able to have my infusion.

In mid-September, I found myself at another appointment with Dr. Farina; we were meeting every few weeks now, it seemed. We talked a lot about what to do. What I needed was an exam under anesthesia (known as an EUA) by a surgeon who could fully assess what was going on inside. My doctor had already put a referral in to his colleague and we were waiting on that, but with huge backlogs on all the wait-lists in Nova Scotia, it was probably going to be a while. I was still waiting for the pelvic ultrasound I'd missed back in May. Dr. Farina wanted to book another flexible sigmoidoscopy since it was almost two years since my last one. He said he was going to talk to his colleagues about my case and pick their brains about whether to increase my medication and whether I should try a different biologic. There were a few different treatments on the market now, though Remicade was the best for everything I had going on. He gave me an emergency prescription for prednisone just in case things got worse, though I knew I would never fill it. I was adamant that I'd never take prednisone again—I'd rather have the surgery.

Three days later, Matt and I woke the girls up before dawn to head to the airport. We were tagging along on Matt's business trip, combining it with a family vacation to Toronto. I didn't feel all that great while we were travelling, but I pushed through and was improving by the end of the day.

Over the next five days we squeezed in as many tourist attractions as we could, planned by the girls who were pumped to be in a big city on vacation. We hadn't travelled outside Atlantic Canada since the pandemic had started, and Rosie didn't remember much about flying to Mexico in 2020 when she was four. We hit up the CN Tower soon after we landed, followed by the aquarium and, over the course of the weekend, the Toronto Zoo, a Blue Jays game, a ferry ride to Centre Island, shopping, brunch, and dinners out, visiting with my brother and with my best friend, Christina, and her family. We spent two nights in a hotel and two nights with my brother. On one of those evenings I had terrible pains, but thankfully as the weekend continued, I felt better.

I was feeling weary by the time my next infusion came in early October. Surprisingly, it made things worse. That evening

I came down with a chill and a low-grade fever. I felt what I often called "infection-y," and whenever that feeling crept up I could tell I had an infection brewing. My body was battling something and suppressing my immune system with Remicade made it worse.

I felt crummy all week and into Thanksgiving weekend. Our friends were hosting a big family party. I almost didn't make it, but in the end dragged myself over with a smile. No one even noticed because I didn't look sick. I could function in pain, and I hid it well. I even made freshly baked pretzels from scratch to contribute to the party. Sure enough, by pushing through (or perhaps with luck), I gradually improved over the next couple of weeks. I had the MRI my doctor had ordered eight months earlier to check on my liver and bile ducts, and everything looked okay.

I was thankful to be improving because I had a birthday coming up—the big four-o—and that week I was feeling good. Wednesday, October 26 was a great day. I was showered with gifts first thing in the morning—among them, a new laptop to finish writing my book. After dropping the girls at school, Matt and I headed off on a morning hike at a nearby ravine, one of my favourite places in the city. I wasn't even bothered when we got caught in the rain for the last ten minutes. We went home to clean up for a lunch out with two of my girlfriends. After a couple of glasses of bubbly, I was off to the spa for a manicure and pedicure, now with a latte in hand. Matt and the girls picked me up afterward, and we were soon on our way for a fancy dinner at a nearby pizzeria. After an amazing day, I still had a big fortieth birthday bash that Matt was planning for the next week to look forward to.

But the very next evening things went off the rails. The pains in my gut were terrible and my belly was making some incredible noises. It sounded like water was gushing around inside, gurgling and growling. I felt really bloated, and out of nowhere, with no nausea, I started vomiting. This brought some relief, but my gut still ached.

We had a busy weekend coming up, so despite my feeble state we bounced from one kids' activity to the next. From a basketball game to a photo session to a running race, I was moving cautiously from one thing to the next, finally dropping one kid at a Halloween party and hosting a play date at home for the other. I snuck away to my room to briefly lie in bed. I spent Sunday hunched at the kitchen table, dutifully stitching a Halloween costume I had yet to finish.

On Halloween night I dragged my butt around the neighbourhood with my kids, their friends, and their friends' moms. Once again, I had a smile on my face. I didn't look sick. I was functioning, though it was a struggle to even stand up straight. Nobody knew. It was a freakishly mild night for the end of October and the moms and I had wine in our travel mugs. The subdivision was bumpin'. I knew I was making terrible choices, but I didn't want to miss out. Why should I have to sit at home sick while everyone else had all the fun? It'd be one thing if I had a contagious stomach bug or a viral illness occasionally. But Crohn's is chronic. My theory was that if I sat out every time I didn't feel well, I'd miss too much, so I never sat out. I also didn't want sympathy—I didn't want to be treated as sickly—so no one but Matt was aware. Even he questioned what I was doing, why I was pushing so hard. I honestly didn't know; I just kept going.

By some stroke of fate, I woke up the next day feeling a little better. Maybe traipsing around the neighbourhood on the hunt for candy had helped straighten things out on the inside? I was feeling some relief, but I still called the helpline at the GI clinic because something was not quite right. I made an appointment to have a call with my doctor the next day.

On Wednesday I stuck the kids in front of the TV after school to ensure I wouldn't be disturbed while I took the call with Dr. Farina. We discussed what to do about these flares I was cycling through. Again, we went over the options. We could try and increase my Remicade to see if that helped, or switch medications altogether. That could make things worse before (or if) they got better. The monthly rounds where he had been planning to present my case to his colleagues had been cancelled in October, so he hadn't had the chance to talk to them. I was still waiting for the ultrasound and surgical consult. In the short term, I could proceed with my regular dose of Remicade as scheduled for the next day. But he decided he wanted to try and book an urgent pelvic MRI, or at least a CT scan, in order to make a more informed decision and determine what the next step—or medication dose—should be. A CT scan would show any infected abscesses (which Remicade could not fix and could, in fact, make worse), and an MRI would highlight fistula tracts (that more Remicade might improve). I hung up so he could make some calls and he phoned me back right away. He had physically walked over to the diagnostic imaging department at the Cobequid Community Health Centre and secured me an appointment for a CT scan on Friday—in two days. If no infected abscesses showed on the CT scan, then we could go ahead with the Remicade. He'd follow up with me by phone on Monday afternoon to discuss the results of the scan, and if the results were positive, I could have my Remicade on Tuesday, possibly at a higher dose. He said if a four-day delay caused issues, we had bigger problems on our hands. I was content with this plan.

The next day I popped over to the radiology department at the hospital to pick up the Gastrografin I'd need to drink before my CT scan. Gastrografin is a contrast agent that contains iodine which is used to highlight the area of the gastrointestinal tract the doctor wants to investigate. The patient is to drink some the night before, some an hour before, and some a few minutes before the scan. While I was out, I ducked into one of my favourite shops to look for an outfit to wear to my birthday party two days later. We'd booked the diner down the street from us and had nearly forty friends and family coming out to celebrate—I couldn't wait. I also couldn't find anything to wear but hoped I'd have luck over the next couple days.

On Friday morning I dropped the girls at school and headed out for the CT scan. I navigated my way to the imaging department, where things moved like clockwork and my name was called in no time. I was wearing leggings, a sports bra, and a sweatshirt so I didn't even have to change into a hospital gown. A friendly technician effortlessly inserted an IV into the back of my hand that would be used to inject more contrast at the time of the scan.

"This shouldn't take long but we'll just see how things look," the tech said as I hopped onto the narrow table that would slide into the ring-shaped scanner. He injected the contrast through my IV and my abdomen was washed in warmth. The machine came to life and a voice guided me through a series of breath-holds as the scanner captured the images.

The tech reappeared at my side. "I just need to call up to the boss. It's looking a little messy in there and they might want to send you over to the emergency department to deal with this."

I balked at this, my suspicions raised. I was feeling all right and I was certain there was no need for that. He came back a few minutes later. His superior had already spoken with Dr. Farina when he'd booked the appointment and knew there was a plan for follow-up on Monday, so he said I was free to go. I stopped at another store on my way home—securing a new shirt for the party. Before I even got home, a call came in from my family doctor's office. She had received the scan results and wanted to make sure there was a follow-up plan. I assured the receptionist my GI doctor was on the case—and by lunchtime he called with the bad news.

He wanted me in the operating room the next day. The scan showed two fistula tracts with a fair bit of fluid and gas built up, and abscesses that needed to be drained. The whole area was inflamed, and further fistulas were branching off in different directions. But as fate would have it, the colorectal surgeon on call in the emergency department that weekend was one of only a few he would trust to do the job right. He'd already discussed it with him and his residents. If I reported to the emergency room the next morning, I'd be assessed, admitted to the hospital directly to general surgery, where I'd have to hope an operating room would become available before the doctor's shift ended at the end of the weekend. Then I'd be put under, the surgeon could poke around to see what was going on, and the abscesses would be drained, all via scope.

"Can't this wait until next week?" I asked, dazed and confused.

"Unfortunately not," came his answer. "Why?"

"Ohhhh, we're supposed to be having my fortieth birthday party tomorrow night," I confessed, my voice wavering. "It's all planned."

He explained that what had been happening to cause me grief was that pus was building in the infected abscesses, and the fistula tracts were likely obstructing and closing over, leading to my pain and bloating. Even my small bowel was now dilating. Receiving Remicade was not recommended due to all the infection. My symptoms were repeatedly escalating and the right guy to fix it was available now. Normally, this could have been scheduled as a regular outpatient procedure but because everything to do with the health system was backed up, it would be ten to twelve weeks before it could be booked. If I tried to wait and do this as an outpatient, it'd be at least a two-to-three-month wait, probably longer. Surgeons were booking eight weeks out *minimum*, and even then, they were only booking procedures related to cancer. I'd continue to cycle through obstructions and fevers while waiting, and it was getting risky.

"This is worth cancelling a party for," he assured me.

As a rule, Dr. Farina has always given me a long leash. He's always been okay to let me wait and see. He has supported me in declining medications I didn't want to take. And he has always tried to help me find solutions.

"I have to put my foot down this time, Heather," he said. I was at risk of a bad infection and a total bowel obstruction if I let this go. Luckily, a surgeon he trusted was on call that weekend. As crappy as it seemed, the stars were actually aligning.

I tried to keep my composure as I jotted down notes. *No food or drink after midnight. Report to ER after 7:00 A.M. shift change. Admit direct to general surgery.* Dr. Farina wished me luck and confirmed we'd still have our follow-up call on Monday afternoon. We hung up and I immediately called Matt, who was driving back from an overnight work trip a few hours away. I couldn't keep my composure any longer. I blurted out the news in one breath through furious tears.

"The CT results are really bad and I need to have surgery and he says I have to go to Emerg tomorrow and we're going to have to cancel my party!" I wailed, bawling now, as all the emotions flooded in—not just about having to cancel the party but about the reality of being so sick. My Crohn's finally had me cornered. I couldn't escape it any longer.

Matt suggested I let my family know right away. He'd call the diner to explain, and once he got back home in a couple of hours, he'd let everyone we'd invited to the party know it was off.

I'd had this disease for nearly twenty-five years but suddenly realized how isolating the past four months had felt—more than ever before. It was no one's fault. I'd been showing up with a smile on my face everywhere I went. I hadn't missed anything—summer trips, family vacations, parties, busy weekends, Halloween. After going to so much effort to push through, showing up happily to everything when everyone was unaware of how I was feeling, it had finally all come crashing down. Earlier that day I'd been shopping for a new outfit to wear to my birthday party, and now I had to cancel the party because I was headed to the OR instead.

Then I felt angry. It was not fair. It wasn't even truly emergency surgery. It was a procedure that could have waited if it had been possible to schedule me as an outpatient through a regular system that was not so dysfunctional. It was great that everything was aligning to deal with it by circumventing the existing system, but seriously?! It shouldn't have to happen that way. Plus, it wasn't simply a cancelled date night, quietly skipping out on plans to hang with friends. The urgency put the spotlight on me; everyone would know something was wrong. I hated it. It felt like my cover had been blown.

I hadn't been trying to hide anything, I just lived in a sort of state of omission. It just wasn't something that came up naturally in conversation—not exactly the kind of thing you casually chit-chat about. Plus, I never wanted to be a downer. My threshold for pain and my tolerance for most any challenge is high. Because I have Crohn's not much can hold me back, but clearly I hadn't even realized that things were…not so good and I'd run out of runway. The situation had been taken out of my control. This treatment may have sounded sudden or extreme to my friends, and rightly so, but this had been brewing. I just hadn't thought it would boil over this way.

Early the next morning, while it was still dark outside, Matt and the girls dropped me off at the entrance to the emergency department. I imagined it was going to be a long day of waiting, so Matt went home to take the kids through their various activities, and I'd keep him posted on my progress. I was triaged right away. There was some confusion over what to do with me when I was called up to be registered. I just kept repeating what my doctor told me. I was to be assessed and admitted through general surgery. I was there to wait for an OR. They were expecting me. After a couple of calls, they seemed to figure it out. I was sent off to wait, hopeful because the emergency department didn't appear to be as slammed as it typically was.

The area was divided into two sections. One side had a sign that said for people with green wristbands only, the other for orange, yellow, and blue wristbands (which seemed to be where all the people who were coughing were sitting, from my observations) but I didn't have any coloured wristband, just the clear one with my personal information. No one had told me where to sit, so I chose a chair in the middle, away from everyone else. There were people who looked miserable, coughing and hacking, and there were those with obvious injuries, sprains or breaks to their arms or legs. Occasionally someone's name was called. Not many more people arrived behind me. I tried to focus on my book. To my relief, I was finally called up after a couple of hours.

A nurse led me into a dingy room that felt more like a cell. There was one stretcher, one garbage can, and a used hospital gown balled up and thrown on the floor. It was cold and I guessed the room hadn't been cleaned between patients. I perched on the stool meant for the staff—there was no way I was touching that stretcher. I was still wearing my winter jacket, balancing my bag on my lap. I was trying not to touch anything.

A surgical resident came in and, since I was on the stool, she sat on the bed to talk with me. I thought it was funny how the tables had been turned. I was pleasantly surprised that she knew my story, my background, and the plan for today. In situations like this, I've always had to repeat my entire history to each new person who entered the room. But she had obviously connected with my GI doctor; her team was expecting me and they were prepared for me. She was friendly and personable, and best of all, she was empathetic. She truly felt bad that I had to be there. I really appreciated that.

Once we'd gone over everything, she left to find a nurse to get me ready. A nurse returned and sent me to the washroom to provide a urine sample; she asked me to meet her back in the hallway. I found her at a chair behind a curtain in the hall, where she efficiently took my blood, conducted the most invasive Covid test I'd ever experienced, and inserted an IV into the back of my hand with ease.

"Did they tell you how long they're going to make you wait before they say, 'Sorry, can't do it today?'" she asked bluntly. Talk about keeping it real.

"I hope it doesn't come to that," I chuckled and smiled meekly back at her.

"Sorry we don't have a room for you. You'll have to wait in the hallway." I peered around the curtain; the hallway was lined with patients waiting, including a guy in handcuffs who was accompanied by a police officer.

"Hang on a second," she said as she disappeared around the corner. She came back in a flash and led me to a much smaller waiting room within the emergency department. There were two couples chatting away; one person from each pair was ill. They'd just met but had all been hanging around since midnight, as I pieced together from their conversation. They carried on gabbing away as if they were just hanging out over coffee, and I wondered why they were in Emerg taking up space. None of them seemed sick enough to be there. But, of course, neither did I.

Someone eventually poked his head in the room to tell me my Covid test had been inconclusive. No doubt, I thought, given that the nurse had bypassed my nasal cavity altogether and swabbed my brain instead. He repeated the test and I waited some more. By 1:00 P.M., just five hours after I arrived, there was a room for me in the hospital. I was surprised, and I felt guilty. All the horror stories I'd been hearing in the news about long wait times and no beds and here I was, sailing right in. But of course, no one needed to spend any time figuring out what was wrong with me or who I should see. I'd already had the CT scan and consulted with doctors.

I hadn't realized I was being admitted into a hospital room. I thought I'd be heading to the OR directly from the ER. I didn't like this; it felt like a hospital stay even though I was just there to cheat the system for a procedure. I declined a wheelchair, and a porter led me on a long, silent walk through the halls of the hospital to my room on 4.1, the general surgery inpatient unit. I was given the bed by the window. I had a roommate, tucked behind her curtains. A nurse checked my vitals and gave me some hospital gowns to change into, one on my front, one on my back as a robe.

I settled onto the bed. All I had with me was my purse, and I slung it with my coat onto the extra chair. It wasn't a terrible place to have to wait; better than the ER. I sent Matt a text to check in. He'd already dropped the girls with our friends for a sleepover and was on his way to meet me at the hospital. I was relieved he could skip the emergency room; we didn't both need to hang out there. He arrived and we sat quietly, both scrolling on our phones. At 3:00 P.M., another porter appeared by the bed. An operating room was available, and the surgeons were ready for me. He whisked both me and my bed away.

After a brief wait in the hallway outside the OR (it felt like we were in a cold, sterile basement), the anesthesiologist asked me what felt like a million questions and then we went over what was going to happen. Then he wheeled my bed into the OR alongside the operating table and I scooched over onto it. I met the surgeon—I'd actually met him before, when he'd helped me out during a previous hospital admission years earlier—and then we had a short consultation. He asked me some questions and we went over what was happening. He said they were going to do a scope to check things out; they would then drain the abscesses inside. They would likely have to put small seton stitches in, which are thin silicone strings (very similar to elastic bands) that are inserted into the fistula tracts to allow them to drain and heal from the inside out.

Then they knocked me out.

"Heather…Heather. We're all done here." I was stirred from a deep slumber by the distant call of my name. I was groggy but starting to come around when I heard a question.

"Hey, aren't you Matt Fegan's wife?"

Huh? I squinted one eye at him. "Yes," I croaked. It was an anesthesiologist (not the one I'd met earlier) and someone, as he explained, who had played soccer with Matt at college. I didn't catch his last name when he introduced himself, but I thought I vaguely remembered him.

My vitals were good, so I was able to skip the recovery room. As he wheeled my bed back to the room, he asked about the kids, who he knew through Matt's Instagram posts. We made small talk while I tried to stay awake; Matt was watching a soccer game on his laptop in my room when we arrived.

"Still always at it, eh?" the anesthesiologist joked. Matt was confused and at first; he had no idea who this guy was because he had a scrub cap on and was wearing a face mask. He pulled his mask down for a moment and it all clicked. They started catching up over soccer, and I drifted back to sleep.

"When can I go home?" I asked when the nurse came to check on me later. I was feeling tired and a little sore, but mostly fine.

"Hopefully tomorrow," she said. "Maybe Monday, since it's the weekend. Depends which doctors are around tomorrow." Umm, no. She was mistaken. If I had my way, I'd be sleeping in my own bed that night. There was no need for me to continue taking up a hospital bed. But I had to wait for the surgeon to follow up. I was starving so Matt grabbed me a bagel and some juice and I ate it with no issues.

Sure enough, when the same friendly surgical resident from that morning came to follow up with me that night, she proved me right. Everything had gone as it was supposed to. I'd see the surgeon for follow-up in four to six weeks, and I would speak with my GI doctor on Monday. She said I could go home, giving me instructions to come back if anything came up.

It was just after 10:00 P.M. as Matt and I headed out to the car. We drove home past the diner where my birthday party was supposed to be taking place right at that very moment.

January 3, 2023

It's a fresh start—a new year—but I'm calling this week my soft launch into 2023. The kids are back in school today after a two-week holiday break, and I'm sitting at my five-hour Remicade infusion. I'll get home just in time for the kids' return. The first two days of the new year have been a magical blend of soaking up the last of the holidays with family—morning coffee by the Christmas tree, cookies, the holiday crossword, finishing a new book—and getting organized, including, finally, on Tuesday evening at the eleventh hour, taking all the Christmas decorations down (there are many—I still love Christmas) and packing them away until next year.

Tomorrow I have an appointment smack-dab in the middle of the morning, leaving not much time to get anything done before I need to crawl through back-to-work city traffic and find parking at the hospital. The appointment at 11:00 A.M. is a follow-up with the surgeon I saw in November. By the time I get home and have lunch, there won't be time to dive too deeply into work before the kids are home from school again. Hopefully I'll then have two solid days of writing under my belt before the weekend hits and I'll be ready to dive into our regularly scheduled programming with a consistent schedule next week—shuttling the kids to their various activities, writing while they're away at school. But I won't entirely count on that because whenever I do, between the kids and myself, someone winds up sick.

Next week will be a doozy because Matt's going away for a week for work. He hasn't been gone for any length of time in years, pre-pandemic at least, and not when we've had two kids in school. Every snack, meal, school run, and dog walk will be on me. Thankfully, I feel well, and after the busy yet somehow-still-relaxing holidays, I feel rested so it shouldn't be a problem. Our Christmas was wonderful—lots of visitors and visiting, late nights and lazy mornings. Best of all, I was healthy.

The procedure in November had gone well. When I followed up with Dr. Farina two days later, he said we'd let things settle and see how it all progressed. The infected abscesses had been fuelling my symptoms, and all the inflammation inside was fuelling the infections, creating that vicious cycle I was in. The hope was it would all heal nicely and I could sink back into the norm I'd experienced through 2020. I'd continue with four-week intervals of Remicade, the seton drains still in place to stop the infectious process and dry out the fistula tracts. My doctor had requested an urgent MRI the same day he'd booked the urgent CT scan. I lucked out with a cancellation and was able to have the pelvic MRI just a few days later. The results were messy, with more fistula tracts lighting up the scan. My ultrasound appointment finally came around again in November (six months after I'd missed it), and there were no problems showing there.

Dr. Farina ordered another flexible sigmoidoscopy because the one in the OR had just been a rigid sigmoidoscopy, covering a much smaller area; he also wanted biopsies, and he wanted to ensure there was no evidence of disease in the small bowel. That appointment came up just a couple of weeks before Christmas. There was, unsurprisingly, significant inflammation in the remaining colon, as usual, but the ileum was normal. No disease in the small bowel. The summary report from that scope read: *At this point I do not feel that increasing the Remicade would lead to significant benefit. I will bring her back in the new year and review consideration of switching biologics.*

Like many, I have high hopes for this year. I'm going to get myself—and our home—organized. There will be major purging, decluttering, and fixing up of neglected areas of the house. I plan to get my health into even better shape through exercise and by cleaning up my diet. My New Year's resolution is to cut back on time wasted on my phone and to read more books, listen to more podcasts, and get outside. I want to raise my profile in preparation for the launch of this book and intend to pitch some accompanying articles to national publications. I'm feeling ready to pick up a new work contract or two.

But all of this depends on my health. Truthfully, I have no idea where that is headed. I've seen it said—in various posts on one motivational Instagram account or another—that living with a chronic illness is a full-time job. I'd never really felt that way about it until the fall of 2022, when managing my Crohn's felt like a full-time gig—juggling appointments, tests, follow-ups, and medications. It seemed like all the appointments ordered for me over the previous year had come up at once in addition to new ones thrown in by my doctor. I had two MRIs, an abdominal ultrasound, a CT scan, the surgical procedure to drain the abscesses, a sigmoidoscopy, plus three in-person and two virtual appointments with Dr. Farina. I'm grateful to have had access to attentive medical care even though the healthcare system is rife with problems and some people are not getting the care they need, sometimes with dire consequences. It sometimes feels as though I have VIP access to the system, having navigated it for nearly twenty-five years.

So last year was a lot, but in many ways the stars aligned to piece together what was going on inside me—the flare like a long, slow burn igniting into a fire that had to be suddenly extinguished.

(We did reschedule the birthday bash by the way, for a couple of weeks after the procedure, and it was a blast.)

Since the surgical procedure to drain the abscesses, I've felt the best I have in a couple of years—not one single pain in my side or obstruction-like symptom in months. What a relief! But as the MRI showed, there are other fistula tracts that aren't abscessed, for now, and what is left of my large bowel is really narrowed, so the prognosis is not great. The situation could escalate at any time. Dr. Farina suggested stopping the long-term antibiotic I'd been on (Cipro) in the new year. I've cautiously done this, and it feels weird and a little risky, although I don't have any signs of infection. I shouldn't be on it forever, so I have to give it a try.

Feeling better also doesn't change the fact that the last five centimetres of my colon are inflamed and diseased, and have been for a long time. It's not entirely wise to leave that in there forever. Will the abscesses and fistulas flare up again? Likely. The sigmoidoscopy in December showed the ileum was normal with no disease into the small bowel, which is great news, but the area below is thickened with significant inflammation. So the next question is, do I switch my medication to try something new to tackle that inflammation? In December, Dr. Farina did not feel that increasing my Remicade would lead to any significant benefit at that point. I'm already on a high and frequent dose of what is probably the best option for my issues. He says we can review and consider switching biologics. Sometimes other drugs do work better for some people. But switching meds could make things worse before they get better and, if the drug fails, we'll be working back up from the bottom of the mountain. Am I thrilled by the idea of traveling down that road again? Not exactly.

In the long term you may require removal of the rectum and a permanent ileostomy, but this will depend on how active your Crohn's is in the future. The long-ago words from my surgeon echo in my head. *The surgery could last you up to twenty years,* he'd predicted. It was far enough in the future that I decided I could deal with that tidbit of information later. That was twenty years ago.

Life is suggesting it may soon be the time to deal with that option, which is to have the surgery, leaving me with a permanent ostomy. There's nothing wrong with having an ostomy. I've had one before. I understand I might have one again. It's just not a decision I feel ready to make given the way I currently feel, right on the brink of better health. If I get sick enough again to warrant surgery (though the doctors say I already warrant surgery…) but sick enough that *I* feel it's warranted, I'll accept it, even welcome it. When my body lets me know it's time, just as Dr. Ste-Marie advised all those years ago—when I can no longer live my life the way I want to—I'll be ready to make the change.

For now, I'm feeling better. I will wait to see what time brings my way—this week, next week, next month, next year. Who knows? These decisions are often taken out of our hands. Maybe a new treatment will calm the inflammation down, so that will be the next conversation to have with my doctor.

IBD is not the worst diagnosis a person can receive; it's not terminal, after all. Crohn's is, by definition, chronic: Persistent. Recurring. Long-lasting. Difficult to eradicate. I'm thankful I'm not always at my worst with my Crohn's disease, but it's *relentless*. I often wonder what it would have been like to not have to deal with any of it. What would the past twenty-five years have been filled with, without all the added turmoil?

But without all of it, I wouldn't have this strength. This grit. This tenacity. I wouldn't truly know suffering. I wouldn't know that I possess the courage to take on another round in this battle and that I have the guts to face whatever life brings—and, oh, these guts of mine!

I may not have all of my *actual* guts anymore, but I am gutsy: courageous, determined, spirited. I believe that sharing openly about living with a debilitating and socially taboo illness like Crohn's takes guts.

So I'm not so sure I'd trade any of the past for a life without Crohn's. This is the life I love, hardships and all. It's a privilege to be able to use the hand I've been dealt to help others and to let them know they are not alone. I dreamed of being a writer long before Crohn's disease came along. Then I grew up to *be* an actual writer. And here I am, writing this for anyone who needs to hear it. I'm happy my story might inspire someone who thinks life can't be lived to the fullest with Crohn's disease or ulcerative colitis.

Because I am living proof it can.

AFTERWORD

My story has continued to evolve, as it always will. After much discussion with Dr. Farina, we decided to increase my dose of Remicade in February 2023. The rationale was to maximize full possible use of the drug before moving on, knowing we'd squeezed every last drop of potential out of the medication. I was doing well, so we thought maybe increasing the drug would give me a boost to make me feel even better. Four infusions later, nothing had changed. I had a follow-up appointment with Dr. Farina at the GI clinic in June.

"How are you feeling?" he asked as he walked into the room.

"I'm feeling good, but I feel like I'm in limbo," I replied.

"Do you want to be in limbo?"

"No, to be honest. I don't."

"Then let's switch your drug."

And just like that, after fourteen years, we decided to bring my time on Remicade to an end. It felt a little like having the rug pulled out from under me. It wasn't the outcome I'd expected heading into that follow-up appointment, though to be honest I don't know what I expected. I realised how much my Remicade infusions had become part of my regular routine, and that they were somewhat of a comfort for me (when they weren't inducing panic attacks disguised as reactions, that is— or maybe it was the other way around).

I was really depending on Remicade, but it was failing me. The drug was keeping my health at baseline—barely—and I deserved better now. It was time to strike, while I was in a decent place health-wise. While I still haven't had any pain or signs of bowel obstruction since the procedure last November, the seton drains are still in place to stop the infectious process, and the fistula tracts have not dried out. Like most everything

I've tried over the years, the procedure got me *just* healthy enough.

Dr. Farina tells me I tolerate too much. We know there is a lot of inflammation in what remains of my diseased colon, and it's been that way for a really long time. He doesn't like the idea of this. He isn't concerned about colon cancer—yet. But what was I waiting for? We know the large bowel is narrowed and the situation could escalate at any time. I'd already been on a high dose of Remicade for a small area of disease. When increasing the dose even higher brought no results, it became clear that Remicade was not going to improve anything any further.

Dr. Farina says patients often cycle through drugs quickly to find what works. Different biologics bring different results to each person. I know deep down this is the right next step. I'm starting Stelara (ustekinumab) right away. It's an easy transition since it's made by the same drug company, and they will continue to provide compassionate coverage of the drug for me.

I worry this switch may make things worse, but what if it makes things better? Stelara works a bit differently than other biologics, in that it targets two naturally occurring proteins, interleukin 12 (IL-12) and IL-23, that contribute to inflammation in the body. The first dose is a two-hour IV infusion, at the same clinic where I received my Remicade, to be followed by a subcutaneous injection every eight weeks. We'll need to wait twelve to sixteen weeks for the full effect (unless I experience drastic changes), at which point we will reassess. I'll need another scope at that point to see if anything's changed inside.

I feel a bit like a living science experiment, but it feels good to be taking action instead of dwelling in limbo. There's another biologic on the list called Entyvio (vedolizumab) I can try next if I need to as I continue on my quest to heal up the inflammation.

All I can do is try.

ACKNOWLEDGEMENTS

To my family, thank you for all your support. Donnie, Debbie, and Denise, thank you for sharing your stories. Mom and Dad, thank you for navigating my chronic illness for me before I could take over for myself, and for all the help in so many ways from the beginning.

Thank you to everyone who gave me moments of their precious time so I could create this book—Dr. Jennifer Jones, Barbara Currie, Jessica Robar, Dr. Michael Vallis, Mallory O'Neill, Shari Smith, Angie Specic, Joseph Windsor, Dr. Kate Lee, and especially Julie Malone—thank you for boldly sharing your journey.

Thank you to Dr. Swift, Dr. Ste-Marie, Dr. Leddin, Dr. Khaliq-Kareemi, and, most especially, Dr. Farina, for your kind and compassionate care over the years. It truly makes a difference and I've been lucky to have you in my corner.

To everyone at Crohn's and Colitis Canada, thank you for the endless work you do to raise awareness and to fight to find a cure.

To everyone at Nimbus, thank you for granting me the amazing opportunity to create this book. This is the guide I wish I'd had when I was diagnosed, and my hope is it will help many people. Thank you for taking a chance on me and this project. It's been a pleasure to work with all of you. To my brilliant editor, Angela Mombourquette, thank you for your expertise and thoughtful feedback. You're amazing at what you do!

Thank you to all the friends who have been there for me, through thick and thin. You know who you are.

Thank you to my girls, Anna and Rosie. You're my greatest

cheerleaders and I am so lucky to be your mom. I'll always love you more, plus one.

Matt, without your support, in every possible way, this book would not have happened. And I would not be living my best life. Thank you for always being here, for your patience, and for always taking care of all of us. I'm forever grateful. I love you more.

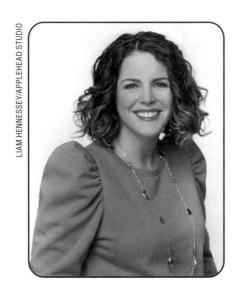

Heather Fegan is a freelance journalist and writer. She is a graduate of the University of King's College School of Journalism. Heather has been a storyteller since age five, regaling her family with "updates" in her own "Heather Chronicles." *Gutsy*, which explores her personal experience of navigating Crohn's Disease over twenty-five years, is her debut book. She lives in Halifax, NS, with her husband and two daughters. Follow her chronicles at heatherfegan.ca and @theheatherchronicles.